Calculating and Reporting Healthcare Statistics

Third Edition

Loretta A. Horton, MEd, RHIA, FAHIMA

AHIMA PRESS

The Web sites listed in this book were current and valid as of the date of publication. However, Web page addresses and the information on them may change or disappear at any time and for any number of reasons. The user is encouraged to perform his or her own general Web searches to locate any site addresses listed here that are no longer valid.

ISBN: 978-1-58426-215-2
AHIMA Product No. AB120709

AHIMA Staff:
Cynthia Douglas, Developmental Editor
Katie Greenock, Editorial and Production Coordinator
Ashley Sullivan, Assistant Editor
Ken Zielske, Director of Publications
Jill Burrington-Brown, RHIA, MS, FAHIMA, Reviewer

AHIMA strives to recognize the value of people from every racial and ethnic background as well as all genders, age groups, and sexual orientations by building its membership and leadership resources to reflect the rich diversity of the American population. AHIMA encourages the celebration and promotion of human diversity through education, mentoring, recognition, leadership, and other programs.

American Health Information Management Association
233 North Michigan Avenue, 21st Floor
Chicago, IL 60601-5800

ahima.org

Contents

About the Author

Loretta A. Horton, MEd, RHIA, received a medical record technician certificate from Research Hospital and Medical Center and a bachelor's degree in psychology from Rockhurst College, both in Kansas City, Missouri; a health information administration post-baccalaureate certificate from Stephens College in Columbia, Missouri; and a master's degree in education, with an emphasis in curriculum and instruction, from Wichita State University in Wichita, Kansas. She also has completed graduate work in sociology at the University of Nebraska in Omaha.

Currently, Loretta is coordinator of the health information technology program and co-chair of the allied health department at Hutchinson Community College in Hutchinson, Kansas. Previously, she worked in a variety of health information settings, including acute care and mental health, and has consulted with long-term care, mental retardation, home health, hospice, and prison systems. Additionally, she has worked as an instructor in the health information administration program at The College of St. Mary in Omaha, Nebraska, and for 3M (Code 3) as a marketing and training coordinator in Salt Lake City.

Loretta has been active in component state organizations as well as the American Health Information Management Association. She has served on the Item Writing Task Force for the Council on Certification and served on the Council on Accreditation. She is a Fellow in the American Health Information Management Association.

She currently lives in Hutchinson, Kansas, with her husband, Bill, who is also a health information professional. She has two daughters, Merritt and Maura.

Acknowledgments

Our thanks to Shannon H. Houser, PhD, MPH, RHIA, assistant professor in the health information management (HIM) program of the department of health services administration at the University of Alabama at Birmingham, for her careful technical review of the text, exercises, and answer key for the third edition of *Calculating and Reporting Healthcare Statistics*, and for creating additional spreadsheet exercises to accompany the textbook.

Also, a word of thanks to the AHIMA Publications staff whose professional work helped to make this textbook a reality. A special thanks to Bill Horton, Becky Hageman, and Christopher Lau, Jill Burrington-Brown, Stephen Sivo, and Lucy Elam, who helped with a review of the textbook, and to Scott Bailey, who contributed to the solutions manual.

Preface

The third edition of *Calculating and Reporting Healthcare Statistics* includes many new exercises and a complete glossary of terms. Terms defined in the glossary appear in bold-face type in the text.

The objectives stated at the beginning of each chapter provide clear and complete explanations of the skills the student should be able to perform, the problems the student should be able to solve, and the terminology the student should be able to define at the conclusion of each chapter.

Calculating and Reporting Healthcare Statistics is designed to introduce statistical computation at the introductory level for use in health information technician (HIT) or health information administration (HIA) education programs, and it follows the curriculum content for these programs. Although intended primarily for students just beginning their health statistics course, this book also can be used by any health professional interested in acquiring knowledge and ability in this area. Moreover, the book may be used, in part, in the assessment of students transferring from a two-year HIT program to a four-year HIA program. Further, it can be used by students taking online classes. Finally, it can serve as a reference or continuing education tool for the experienced HIM practitioner.

The book is divided into thirteen chapters. Each chapter contains instructional sections, most of which provide a definition or formula, explanatory material, and examples. Most chapters contain exercises that test the student's comprehension of the material. The chapters also offer tests that can be used to evaluate student progress. The book also provides assignments for compiling inpatient service days; average length of stay and occupancy; data presentation; and computerization of statistics. Finally, the book includes three appendices. Appendix A contains all the formulas studied in the chapters; appendix B is a glossary of the terminology on which the statistical formulas are based; and—new to this edition—appendix C contains the answers to odd-numbered chapter exercises.

Throughout the text, a number of figures and tables display samples of statistical reports from the "real world" of health information management. Their inclusion in the book has a specific purpose. The real world often does not mimic the classroom. Facilities sometimes have sets of rules that may not be exactly like those taught in classrooms and often change.

HIM practitioners may be asked to produce an almost limitless number of rates from data collection. However, as an introduction to the field, this book discusses only those healthcare statistics that HIM professionals compute most often. Moreover, the book focuses on commonly used rates and percentages computed principally on hospital inpatients. However, the author also has included non–acute care data and examples. Therefore, when a definition or formula states patient, it also could mean client, member, or resident.

Chapter 1, Introduction to Health Statistics, defines statistics and discusses the reasons for studying them. It also explains the sources of statistics in the healthcare setting and the many ways that healthcare statistics are used.

Chapter 2, Mathematics Review, defines the basic mathematics terms used in healthcare settings and provides illustrations showing how they are used in calculations. The terms discussed include fractions, quotients, decimals, ratio, proportion, rates, percentages, and rounding.

Chapter 3, Patient Census Data, describes the different types of census taken in healthcare settings and how to calculate and report each type. The basic types of census discussed include inpatient census, complete master census, daily inpatient census, and inpatient service days.

Chapter 4, Percentage of Occupancy, addresses bed occupancy and bed turnover rate in the healthcare setting. The chapter defines many of the different terms used in calculating such percentages and illustrates how the percentages are computed.

Chapter 5, Length of Stay, explains the terms used to characterize the different types of length of stay in a healthcare setting, including total length of stay, average length of stay, and leave of absence days. The chapter also illustrates how the different types of length of stay are calculated.

Chapter 6, Death (Mortality) Rates, defines the different types of death rates that are computed in the healthcare setting, including gross, net, postoperative, anesthesia, maternal, infant, fetal, and cancer mortality rates. The formula used to calculate each type of death rate is provided, along with sample calculations.

Chapter 7, Hospital Autopsies and Autopsy Rates, discusses autopsies and coroner's cases. Formulas are included for the gross autopsy rate, net autopsy rate, adjusted hospital autopsy rate, newborn autopsy rate, and fetal autopsy rate. Examples clarify how each rate is computed.

Chapter 8, Morbidity and Other Miscellaneous Rates, discusses nosocomial and postoperative infection rates and how they are calculated. The chapter also covers C-section and consultation rates, and presents a general formula for calculating other rates.

Chapter 9, Statistics Computed within the Health Information Management Department, focuses on the common, everyday computations made by health information management staff. The discussion touches on the use of statistics to calculate unit cost, productivity, and staffing levels. Various computerized reports, including discharge, financial, readmission rate, and case-mix index reports, are discussed.

Chapter 10, Descriptive Statistics in Healthcare, focuses on rank, quartile, decile, and percentile and how and why percentiles are used. Measures of central tendency are reviewed such as the mean, median, mode and range, variance, and standard deviation.

Chapter 11, Presentation of Data, explores different types of data and their presentation tools. The different types of categorical data are defined, and the most effective ways to display data are illustrated.

Chapter 12, Inferential Statistics in Healthcare, is designed with the four-year health information administration student in mind. It describes how to interpret the standard error of the mean and confidence intervals. The null hypothesis is explained along with the importance of t tests, ANOVA, and chi square. This chapter is not designed to take the place of a student's statistics course but, rather, to provide a review of concepts.

Chapter 13, Basic Research Principles, covers basic information about research and the different types of research, focusing on the difference between quantitative and qualitative research. It also discusses research design and the steps in the research process, explains various data collection techniques, and addresses how to select study samples, analyze data, and draw conclusions. Additionally, it covers the Institutional Review Board and its role in research.

In many healthcare facilities, most data are generated electronically. Nevertheless, it is still important that health information practitioners understand the concepts of healthcare statistics.

Note to educators: Instructor materials for this book include lesson plans, chapter slides, a full solutions manual for all exercises and chapter tests, and other useful resources. The instructor materials are available in online format through the Assembly on Education (AOE) Community of Practice (CoP). Instructors who are AHIMA members can sign up for this private community by clicking on the help icon within the CoP home page and requesting additional information on becoming an AOE CoP member. An instructor who is not an AHIMA member or an AHIMA member who is not an instructor may contact the publisher at publications@ahima.org. The instructor materials are not available to students enrolled in college or university programs.

Chapter 1
Introduction to Health Statistics

Objectives

At the conclusion of this chapter, you should be able to:

- Define statistics
- Appreciate the need to study healthcare statistics
- Differentiate between descriptive and inferential statistics
- Recognize where statistics in healthcare originate
- Identify the users of healthcare statistics

Statistics

The term *statistic* refers to a number computed from a larger collection of numbers which collectively constitute a sample of data (for instance, the mean or the average value of a variable belonging to a sample of data). A sample is a small part (a subset) of a larger group of data (a population). The term *statistics* is more broadly defined as a branch of mathematics concerned with collecting, organizing, summarizing, and analyzing data.

Origins of the Term

Originally, the term *statistics* referred to the collection of information about and for the "state." The word comes from the Italian word *stato,* meaning "state." One need only think of our own government and its statistics-collecting organizations, such as the Bureau of Labor Statistics, the National Center for Health Statistics (NCHS), the Administration on Aging, the Centers for Disease Control and Prevention (CDC), the Centers for Medicare and Medicaid Services (CMS), and so on.

Reasons for Studying Statistics

Statistics is really about decision making. In every area of our lives, we are expected to make decisions. To do that, we must have some information. Because information is often incomplete in healthcare settings, we must learn to estimate the characteristics of a complete population using statistics.

All organizations keep statistics in order to make decisions about their business. For example, an organization may use statistics to determine its markets, that is, to identify who is using its services and how it can increase those services. Libraries need information on what the public is reading in order to satisfy public interest and needs. Educational institutions need statistics about types of employment that students can get after graduation in order to improve the curriculum for future students.

In the healthcare industry, there are compelling reasons to collect and analyze data. For example, statistics kept on activities in the healthcare facility indicate why patients come to the facility and the costs of taking care of them. Patient care statistics and studies on performance can show the quality of care provided. Many accrediting agencies require a data analysis system as part of accreditation, and many third-party payers require facilities to collect performance data. Administrators also may use statistics for prioritizing needed services and to point to areas where efficiency and effectiveness might be increased. Additionally, healthcare facilities are interested in the types of patients they have with respect to their diagnoses in order to maintain the optimum physician specialty mix they need.

The government also needs to maintain statistics on and about the population in order to provide services. For example, the CDC is recognized as the lead agency responsible for protecting the health of the United States population by providing credible information to help individuals make the right healthcare decisions.

To obtain the knowledge they need, organizations first must have data. Data are unprocessed facts and figures that can be deliberately selected, processed, and organized to provide useful information. This leads, in turn, to facts, which are pieces of information representing the truth. And facts lead to an improved understanding of the original, unprocessed information. Improved understanding gives individuals the power to make better decisions. The sequence, then, is as follows:

Data → Information → Facts → Improved understanding → Better decision making

Health statistics provide information about the health of people and their utilization of healthcare services. Examples of healthcare statistics include average longevity, birth rates, death rates, incidence of a particular disease in a state or the United States as a whole, and the frequency of usage of a particular type of service within a hospital.

Other common uses of statistics may include divorce rates in a country, accident rates in a state, crime statistics in a city, percent of HIV carriers in the world, and even the standings of candidates in a political race. To serve each of these and many other purposes, the figures used in the statistics must be relevant and reliable. "To be relevant" refers to the applicability of the statistics. "To be reliable" means that there is some consistency of results. For example, if your instructor graded a test and then asked another instructor to grade the same test and they both had the same results, the results could be said to be reliable.

Descriptive Statistics versus Inferential Statistics

The primary focus of descriptive statistics is to organize and describe the features of data in a study. **Descriptive statistics** describe what the data show about the characteristics of a sample. For example, we may need to know the average age of our patients or which service is used most in our facility. Both these statistics are used to describe data. **Inferential statistics,** on the other hand, help us make inferences or guess about a larger group of data by drawing conclusions from a small group of data. The smaller group of data is often called a sample, which is a portion of the larger group, or population. The results obtained from the sample, if gathered carefully, are assumed to be typical of the entire population.

Sources of Healthcare Statistics

Healthcare information is derived from both primary and secondary data sources. Statistics usually come from a primary data source, or firsthand documents. In healthcare, *primary data source* refers to the health record that was developed by healthcare professionals in the process of providing care. *Secondary data sources* are data from a source other than the primary sources. Secondary data sources are facility-specific. For example, the disease and operation index is a secondary source of information. All the information in the index comes from a primary data source—the health record. Registries are also considered secondary data sources. For example, information from the medical record may be used to create a cancer or trauma registry.

The health record is one of the most important primary sources of health statistics because it contains most of the health facts about patients.

Another source of health information is the census. A **census** is defined as a count of a particular population. The U.S. government conducts a census, that is, a count of the people residing in the United States and their location. This kind of census is called a population census. "Census" comes from the Latin word *censere,* which means "to assess or to tax." The Romans started taking a census in order to make a register of the people and their property. One reason was to identify individuals who could serve in their armies and another was to place a value on their property so they could be taxed.

The U.S. Constitution requires that a population census be taken every 10 years. The main reason is to determine the number of Congressional representatives in the states. Over the years, Congress has authorized gathering more information about each person. The census now is used in many ways. For instance, the amount of government monies given to school districts is based partly on the number of children in a particular district. Congress also has requested that other types of censuses be taken periodically. These include a census of the types of businesses and industries in the U.S., for example, farms and fisheries, construction, foreign trade, manufacturing, and energy companies. All census information is available to the public.

Healthcare facilities also have a census, which is the count of patients present at a specific time and in a particular place. In **hospitals,** this is referred to as the **inpatient census.** The hospital census is a source of primary information. **Ambulatory care** facilities also may keep a census. This figure usually represents the number of **visits** or encounters during a specified period, usually one day. An **encounter** is defined in appendix B of this book as the direct personal contact between a patient and a physician or other person authorized by state licensure and, if applicable, by medical staff bylaws to order or furnish healthcare services for the diagnosis or treatment of the patient.

Hospital departments also keep statistics on the activities they perform for patients. For example, the laboratory department may keep data on the number of lab tests performed on **inpatients** and **outpatients.** The radiology department may keep track of the number of chest and hip x-rays. The physical therapy department may use statistical information such as the number of patient visits in deciding whether to hire additional physical therapists or add physical therapist assistants to their staff. These reports may be used in turn by the managers of the departments for productivity reports and combined to produce a report of activity for the entire facility. The administration of your hospital might ask you to keep data on the number of patients transferred to another hospital for a cardiac catheterization in order to determine the need for that service at your facility.

Another example of a primary source of information is **vital statistics.** The National Vital Statistics System (NVSS) is part of the National Center for Health Statistics (NCHS) of the Centers for Disease Control and Prevention (CDC). These data are provided throughout the 50 states, Washington, D.C., New York City, and five territories of the United States (Puerto Rico, the Virgin Islands, Guam, American Samoa, and the Commonwealth of the Northern Mariana Islands) to the NCHS. *Vital statistics* refers to a special group of statistics that record important events in our lives such as birth, marriage, death, divorce, and fetal deaths. Healthcare facilities are interested in births and deaths, fetal deaths, and induced terminations of pregnancy and generally are responsible for completing certificates for births, fetal deaths, abortions, and, occasionally, death certificates. All states have laws that require this information. The certificates are reported to the individual state registrars and maintained permanently.

The NCHS has developed standard forms and procedures that states and territories must use to ensure consistent collection of data. Forms and instructions are usually updated about every 10 years; the last revision to the birth, death, and fetal death certificates was in 2003.

Data from the states and territories provide information for use in medical research and are extremely valuable in estimating population growth in particular areas of the country and essential in planning and evaluating maternal and child health programs. NCHS prepares and publishes national statistics based on vital statistics data because they are important in the fields of social welfare and public health.

Users of Health Statistics

All organizations concerned with healthcare collect and use statistics. Following are examples of individuals and organizations that collect statistics and how they use statistics:

- Healthcare Administration: Inpatient facilities use health statistics to help address staffing issues and to determine the types of services to provide. For example, if the number of patients in the intensive care unit is increasing, the hospital administration may want to consider adding beds and staff to meet the growing need. Conversely, if a request is made to the hospital administration for new facilities and equipment that cannot be substantiated by the statistics, it is unlikely the request will be granted.

- Healthcare Department Managers: Individual department managers in healthcare organizations use statistics to implement their department goals. For example, a manager needs to know if he or she is staying within budget. If not, the manager will need to investigate the reason.

- Cancer Registries: A cancer registry may be maintained by a separate department or may be a function of the health information department. States may also have a state cancer registry that is responsible for collecting data about cancer. A cancer registry collects data about the diagnosis, treatment, and follow-up of cancer patients. These statistics are important in tracking cancer survival rates. Facilities may choose to undergo accreditation through the American College of Surgeons. This is an evaluation by an independent team to determine whether or not the facility's Cancer Registry meets their standards. Statistics must show the facility is providing high-quality care and follow-up to its cancer patients.

- **Nursing Facilities:** Long-term care facilities may use statistics to determine the types of payers their patients have. These statistics also are helpful in demonstrating to the public the types of patients being cared for.

- **Home Health (HH):** Home health agencies provide care to elderly, disabled, and/or convalescent patients in their homes. These agencies keep statistics to determine the types of services used by their patients and their outcomes. For example, a home health agency would need to know the number of nursing visits, home health aide visits, physical therapy treatments, and patients with various types of equipment such as oxygen machines or other respiratory aids. Additionally, agencies will report patient outcomes, such as, the number of patients who have improved, the number of patients who were compliant with taking their medications, or the number of patients who had to be readmitted to a hospital.

- **Hospice:** Hospice programs provide care and psychosocial support to terminally ill patients and their families. These services may be given in either the home or an inpatient setting. A hospice needs to know types of illnesses in order to match the appropriate caregiver with each patient.

- Mental Health Facilities: These may be inpatient or outpatient facilities. These facilities use health statistics to determine whether they are providing the proper services for patients in the community.

- Drug and Alcohol Facilities: These programs may be inpatient, ambulatory, or a combination of the two. Statistics are important in this area to show the success rates of these facilities' clients.

- Outpatient Facilities: These include physician clinics, surgery centers, emergency centers, and the like. Outpatient facilities often use statistics to determine whether they are providing the proper level of care to the community.

- **Managed Care Organizations (MCOs):** MCOs use statistics to determine whether they are providing the correct level of care at the best cost. Additionally, MCOs contract with healthcare facilities to provide specific services to their members at a particular cost. The MCO pays the agreed upon amount each time a member uses the service. Typically, the MCO receives a discounted rate and this results in individual members of the MCO paying less out of pocket.

- Healthcare Researchers: Researchers depend on healthcare statistics to perform **research.** Some examples include research in managed care, health law and regulations, mergers and acquisitions of healthcare facilities, physician practice issues, different types of illness and risk factors, telehealth issues, pharmaceutical research, and so on.

- Accreditation Agencies: These organizations use healthcare statistics to determine the most common diagnoses and procedures and whether the resources are available to treat patients with those diagnoses.

- Federal Government: The U.S. government collects information for public health issues. For example, the CDC reports data on births, deaths, birth defects, cancer, HIV/AIDS, just to name a few of the categories of data.

Handy Tip: Health information management (HIM) practitioners must remember that, first and foremost, statistics must be gathered and formulated, or expressed in systematic terms or concepts, before they even exist. HIM practitioners are usually the individuals who gather and formulate this information.

Because HIM practitioners have a broad knowledge of healthcare facilities as well as immediate access to a wide range of clinical data, they are in the best position to collect, prepare, analyze, and interpret healthcare data. HIM practitioners must learn acceptable terminology, definitions, and computational methodology if they are to provide the basic and most frequently used health statistics.

Chapter 1 Test

Select the best answer to the following questions:

1. Which of the following is the lead agency responsible for protecting the health of the U.S. population?
   a. Centers for Disease Control and Prevention
   b. Department of Health and Human Services
   c. Food and Drug Administration
   d. Environmental Protection Agency

2. Which of the following are unprocessed facts and figures?
   a. Numbers
   b. Data
   c. Statistics
   d. Knowledge

3. A piece of information representing the truth is called which of the following?
   a. A fact
   b. Data
   c. A statistic
   d. Improved understanding

4. Health statistics provide information about the health of which of the following?
   a. Terminally ill patients
   b. Healthcare employees
   c. Family practice physicians
   d. The population in general

5. Which of the following is considered a source of primary data?
   a. The master patient index
   b. The card catalog
   c. The health record
   d. The Department of Health and Human Services

6. A census is defined as which of the following?
   a. A collection of data
   b. A survey conducted with a small group
   c. A bureau of research specialists
   d. A count of a particular population

(continued on next page)

Chapter 1 Test (continued)

7. What is the term given to describe the count of patients present at a specific time and in a particular place in a hospital setting?
   a. An inpatient census
   b. A diagnosis-related group
   c. A case-mix report
   d. A DRG category

8. What are statistics called that refer to important events in our lives, such as births, marriages, deaths, and divorces?
   a. Health statistics
   b. Vital statistics
   c. Human statistics
   d. Popular statistics

9. Which of the following is a single item or datum calculated from and representing a collection of items?
   a. A sample
   b. Data
   c. A statistic
   d. A fact

Indicate whether the following statements are true or false:

10. Statistics can be one piece of data or a quantity of data.

11. Data are facts and/or figures that are deliberately selected and processed.

12. The primary reason to keep statistics is for decision making.

13. Third-party payers are not really interested in healthcare statistics.

14. Data are the same thing as information.

15. A diabetes registry is an example of a primary data source.

Chapter 2
Mathematics Review

Objectives

At the conclusion of this chapter, you should be able to:

- Explain fraction, quotient, decimal, ratio, proportion, rate, and percentage
- Understand the difference between a numerator and denominator
- Understand how to round whole numbers and decimals
- Convert fractions and decimals to percentages
- Understand how to average a group of numbers

Review of Basic Mathematical Expressions

Numbers may be expressed in a variety of ways for use in calculating statistics. The following sections discuss fractions, how to round numbers, percentages, ratios, rates, and averages.

Fractions

A **fraction** is one or more parts of the whole. Figure 2.1 shows two circles; the first circle is split into two equal parts, and the second shows one part of the circle larger than the other part. The fraction of the first circle is $\frac{1}{2}$; the fraction of the second circle (in darker color) is $\frac{3}{4}$. The top number is called the **numerator** and the bottom number is called the **denominator.**

> **Example:** Of the 40 patients with diabetes seen last month in a physician's clinic, 20 were Caucasian, 10 were African-American, and 10 were Asian-American. The following fractions show the number of patients of each race compared to the total number of patients who visited the clinic: Caucasian, $\frac{20}{40}$; African-American, $\frac{10}{40}$; and Asian-American, $\frac{10}{40}$. Fractions should be converted to their simplest form. Each fraction can be converted by dividing both top (numerator) and bottom (denominator) by a common factor. In this example, both the numerator and the denominator can be divided by 10: Caucasians, $\frac{2}{4}$; African-American, $\frac{1}{4}$; and Asian-American $\frac{1}{4}$. The first fraction can be further simplified with the common factor of 2; thus, $\frac{2}{4}$ can be expressed as $\frac{1}{2}$.

Exercise 2.1

Find the simplest form of each of the following fractions:

1. $\dfrac{40}{80}$

2. $\dfrac{3}{9}$

3. $\dfrac{75}{150}$

4. $\dfrac{6}{36}$

5. $\dfrac{20}{100}$

Quotient

A **quotient** is the number obtained by dividing the numerator of a fraction by the denominator. This number may be expressed in **decimals**.

Figure 2.1.   Fractions of a Circle

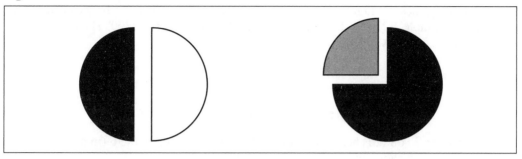

Example: The 14 members of your health information class decide to participate in your college's information day. The booth is going to be open for 21 hours over a three-day period. To find out how many hours each student would need to attend to the booth, you would divide the numerator (21 hours) by the denominator (14 students). This calculation gives a quotient of 1.5. Thus, each student would have to attend the booth for 1.5 hours.

Decimal Fraction

Decimal fractions are simply referred to as decimals. The notation indicates a value that is less than one. In 14.37, for example, the digits to the right of the decimal point (3 and 7) are called decimal digits. The decimal point is used to separate the fraction of a **whole number** (.37) from the whole number itself (14). The decimal point is not ordinarily used in whole numbers (for example, 14.0) unless the healthcare facility has a particular reason for doing so.

Handy Tip: The decimal .5 is usually written as 0.5 in order to call attention to the decimal point.

Rounding Numbers

Rounding is a process of approximating a number. Numbers may be rounded to the nearest 10, 100, and so on.

Rounding to the Nearest Ten

Rounding to the nearest ten means that any number between multiples of ten (10, 20, 30, 40, and so on) is rounded to the multiple it is closest to. For example, 31 falls between 30 and 40 but is closer to 30, so it is rounded to 30. However, 37 is closer to 40, so it is rounded to 40. When a number is exactly between the two multiples of ten, the rule of thumb is to round up. Thus, 35 would be rounded up to 40 as in the example below.

Rounding to the Nearest Hundred

Rounding to the nearest hundred refers to rounding numbers that fall between multiples of 100. For example, 327 falls between 300 and 400 but is closer to 300. Thus, the 2 in the tens place indicates that 327 should be rounded down to 300.

3	2	7
↓	↓	↓
hundreds	tens	ones

The number 7,868 falls between 7,800 and 7,900. In this case, the 6 (in the tens place) indicates that 7,868 should be rounded up to 7,900.

7	8	6	8
↓	↓	↓	↓
thousands	hundreds	tens	ones

Rounding Decimals

Most healthcare statistics are reported as decimals, and each healthcare facility has its own policy on the number of decimal places to be used in computing and reporting percentages. The principles that apply to rounding whole numbers also apply to rounding decimals. To round to the nearest whole number, look at the first digit to the right of the decimal point (tenths); if the number is 5 or more, the whole number should be rounded up; if the number is less than 5, the whole number should be left as it is. Thus, the whole number in 14.4 should remain at 14; however, 14.5 should be rounded up to 15.

To round to the nearest tenth, you do the same thing except use the hundredths digit rather than the tenths. The hundredths is the second digit to the right of the decimal point. For example, 14.46 would be rounded up one to 14.5 because the 6 in .46 is greater than 5. In the case of 14.13, the 3 in .13 is less than 5, so the .1 is kept rather than rounding up. To round to the nearest hundredths, the calculation must be carried out to three decimal places (the thousandths digit) and then rounded. For example, 14.657 would be rounded up to 14.66 because the 7 in .657 is greater than 5. In the case of 14.654, the 4 in .654 is less than 5, so the .65 is kept rather than rounding up.

> **Handy Tip:** When the decimal points must be carried out to two places, the calculation should be carried out to one more place in the quotient and rounded back. For example:
>
> $$\frac{1}{7} = 0.14286 = 14.29\%; \; or$$
>
> $$1 \times \frac{1}{7} = 14.286 = 14.29$$

Exercise 2.2

Round to two decimal places.
Find the quotient in the following fractions.

1. $\dfrac{3}{5}$

2. $\dfrac{8}{12}$

3. $\dfrac{34}{56}$

4. $\dfrac{107}{98}$

5. $\dfrac{545}{654}$

Exercise 2.3

Round the following numbers to the nearest ten.

1. 48

2. 356

3. 311

4. 5,896

5. 3,258

6. 9,631

7. 232,563

8. 2,634

9. 48,605

10. 8,563

Round the following numbers to the nearest hundred.

11. 651

12. 123

13. 8,307

14. 7,534

15. 5,781

(continued on next page)

Exercise 2.3 (continued)

Round to the nearest whole number.

16. 18.3

17. 32.5

18. 23.1

19. 152.6

20. 99.4

Round to one decimal place.

21. 15.89

22. 18.58

23. 32.62

24. 99.98

25. 124.07

Percentage

The ratio of a part to the whole is often expressed as a **percentage.** A percentage is a fraction expressed in hundredths. Percent means "per 100." There is a specific way to write this. For example, .34 would be written as $\frac{34}{100}$ and is equal to 34%.

Percentages are a useful way to make fair comparisons. For example, if 20 patients died in hospital A last month and 50 patients died in hospital B during the same period, one might conclude that it would be better to use the services at hospital A because hospital A had fewer deaths. However, that conclusion would be wrong if hospital A had 100 discharges during the month and hospital B had 500 discharges for the same period.

Not all percentages are converted to whole numbers. For example:

$$\frac{1}{8} = .125 = 12.5\%$$

Changing a Fraction to a Percentage

To change a fraction to a percentage, divide the numerator by the denominator and multiply by 100. For example, to change $\frac{1}{2}$ to a percentage, divide 1 by 2 and multiply by 100. The calculation is as follows:

$$\frac{1}{2} = 0.5 \times 100 = 50\%$$

Changing a Decimal to a Percentage

To change a decimal to a percentage, simply multiply the decimal by 100. The calculation changes the position of the decimal point. For example:

$$0.29 \times 100 = 29\%$$

Changing a Percentage to a Fraction

To convert a percentage to a fraction, eliminate the percent sign and multiply the number by $\frac{1}{100}$. A simpler version of this is to place the number in the numerator and 100 in the denominator. For example:

$$5\% \text{ would be } 5 \times \frac{1}{100} = \frac{5}{100}$$

$$15\% \text{ would be } 15 \times \frac{1}{100} = \frac{15}{100}$$

Fractions are usually converted to their simplest form. In the example of 5%, both 5 and 100 can be divided by 5, which would result in a fraction of $\frac{1}{20}$. In the example 15%, again, both 15 and 100 are divisible by 5, resulting in a fraction of $\frac{3}{20}$.

Changing a Percentage to a Decimal

To convert a percentage to a decimal, eliminate the percent sign and place a decimal point two places to the left. If the percentage is only one digit, place a 0 in front of it and place the decimal point in front of the 0. For example:

$$76\% \text{ would be } 0.76$$

$$4\% \text{ would be } 0.04$$

$$104\% \text{ would be } 1.04$$

Exercise 2.4

Complete the following conversions.

Fractions to percentages:

1. $\frac{3}{4}$

2. $\frac{4}{5}$

3. $\frac{7}{8}$

4. $\frac{9}{10}$

5. $\frac{1}{15}$

(continued on next page)

Exercise 2.4 (continued)

Decimals to percentages:

  6. 0.75

  7. 0.09

  8. 0.16

  9. 0.325

10. 0.965

Percentages to fractions:

11. 35%

12. 82%

13. 25%

14. 4%

15. 33%

Percentages to decimals:

16. 17%

17. 3%

18. 0.5%

19. 118%

20. 99%

Ratio

Three general classes of mathematical parameters are used to relate the number of cases, diseases, patients, or outcomes in the healthcare environment to the size of the source population in which they occur. The most basic measure is the **ratio.** A ratio expresses the relationship of one quantity to another.

Calculating Ratio

To calculate a ratio, one quantity is divided by another. The number can be greater than 1 or less than 1. For example, if seven men and five women were in a group, the ratio of men to women would be $\frac{7}{5}$. This ratio also may be written as 7:5 and verbalized as 7 to 5. The numbers 7 and 5 have no common factors, so this ratio cannot be simplified. However, if the group consisted of 6 men and 10 women, for example, the ratio would be 6:10. Because the numbers in this ratio have a common factor of 2, the ratio can be simplified by dividing each number by 2, which simplifies the ratio to 3:5.

$$\text{Ratio: } \frac{x}{y} = \frac{6}{10}$$

or

$$\text{Ratio: } \frac{y}{x} = \frac{10}{6}$$

Exercise 2.5

Express the following ratios in their simplest form.

1. 14:28
2. 3:12
3. 5:10
4. 7:49
5. 1:16

Proportion

A **proportion** is a type of ratio in which x is a portion of the whole $(x + y)$. In a proportion, the numerator is always included in the denominator. For example, if two women out of a group of ten over the age of 50 have had breast cancer, where $x = 2$ (women who have had breast cancer) and $y = 8$ (women who have not had breast cancer), the calculation would be 2 divided by 10. The proportion of women that have breast cancer is 0.2.

$$\frac{x}{(x+y)} = \frac{2}{(2+8)} = 0.2$$

Rate

A **rate** is a ratio in which there is a distinct relationship between the numerator and denominator and the denominator often implies a large base population. A measure of time is often an intrinsic part of the denominator. Healthcare facilities calculate many types of rates in order to determine how the facilities are performing.

Handy Tip: Misplaced decimal points can result in mathematical errors. All calculations should be checked for sensible answers. For example, a hospital death rate of 25 percent should seem unreasonable because it indicates that one of every four patients treated at this hospital died. Why would anyone want to be treated at a hospital that had a 25 percent death rate? Thus, the decimal placement in this calculation should be checked. The correct death rate for this hospital may be 2.5 percent or .25 percent, which would be more realistic.

The term *rate* is often used loosely to refer to rate, proportion, percentage, and ratio. Indeed, many books and organizations use these terms interchangeably. For this reason, it is important to be aware of how any measure being reported has actually been defined and calculated.

Calculating Rate

The basic rule of thumb for calculating rate is to indicate the number of times something *actually* happened in relation to the number of times it *could have* happened (actual/potential). For example, let's say you have been eating out often in the past few weeks. To calculate the rate of meals you have eaten out in one week, divide the number of meals that were eaten out (for example, 13) by the number of meals you could have eaten out (21). The rate is $\frac{13}{21}$, or 61.9 percent. The formula for determining rate is as follows:

$$Rate = \frac{Part}{Base}, \text{ or } R = \frac{P}{B}$$

Table 2.1 shows the equations for calculating ratio, proportion, percentage, and rate.

Table 2.2 shows a sample computerized statistical report provided by the information systems (IS) department of an acute care facility and illustrates how the department uses percentages.

Handy Tip: Everyone has heard this saying about computers: "garbage in, garbage out," or "GIGO." Computers are great for many things, including performing statistical calculations, but they must be programmed accurately to calculate correctly. Even the function of rounding needs to be validated. For example, it is not unheard of for an IS manager to ask a health information management (HIM) professional for the formula for death rate because the computer system crashed and all new formulas and specifications had to be reprogrammed.

Table 2.1.   Review of Equations for Calculating Ratio, Proportion, Percentage, and Rate

The following list of equations differentiates among ratio, proportion, percentage, and rate, where $x = 5$ men and $y = 3$ women.

Ratio: $\dfrac{x}{y} = \dfrac{5}{3}$

Proportion: $\dfrac{x}{(x + y)} = \dfrac{5}{(5 + 3)}$

Percentage: $\left[\dfrac{x}{(x + y)}\right] \times 100 = \left[\dfrac{5}{(5 + 3)}\right] \times 100$

Rate: $R = \dfrac{Part}{Base} \text{ or } R = \dfrac{P}{B}$

Table 2.2.   Administrator's Semiannual Reference Report

Administrator's Semiannual Reference Report Admissions by Day of Week 1/1/20XX–6/30/20XX		
Day	**Number of Patients**	**Percent of Patients**
Sunday	1,187	19.1
Monday	755	11.3
Tuesday	1,085	16.3
Wednesday	1,031	15.5
Thursday	1,024	17.0
Friday	808	12.1
Saturday	773	11.6
Total	**6,663**	**100.0**

Averages

An average is the value obtained by dividing the sum of a set of numbers by the number of values. Average is generally referred to as the arithmetic mean to distinguish it from the mode or median. (This is covered in more detail in chapter 10.)

The symbol $\overline{X}$ (pronounced "ex bar") is used to represent the mean in this formula.

$$\frac{Sum\ of\ all\ the\ values}{Number\ of\ all\ the\ values\ involved} = \overline{X}$$

Example: Let's say that you have taken six medical terminology tests. Your scores are 82, 78, 94, 56, 91, and 85. Adding together the scores gives you a total score of 486. Now, divide this by 6 (the number of tests you have taken). This equals 81. This means that your average score on the medical terminology tests is 81.

Chapter 2 Test

Complete the following exercises.

1. Convert the fraction $\frac{1}{5}$ to a quotient and then a percentage.

2. Round the following percentages to two decimal places.
   a. 15.894%
   b. 13.256%
   c. 0.765%
   d. 0.068%
   e. 56.325%

3. Convert $\frac{1}{6}$ to a percentage to two decimal points.

(continued on next page)

Chapter 2 Test (continued)

4. Review table 2.2 to verify that the calculations are correct. Note that the percent of patients listed in this report is the actual/potential.

$$\left(\frac{Actual\ \#\ of\ patients}{Potential\ \#\ of\ patients}\right) \times 100$$

5. It was reported in your department meeting that over the past year your hospital increased the number of employees by 12 percent. Last year there were 347 people employed, how many are employed this year? (Round to a whole number.)

6. Your manager needs to purchase a personal computer for the new receptionist in your department. The usual price is $1,100. The local supply company gives the facility an 11.5 percent reduction on all items they purchase. What price will your manager pay?

7. Your beginning salary as an analyst in the HIM department is $12.50 per hour. You are due to receive a 3.5 percent cost-of-living raise in your next paycheck. Your performance evaluation is coming up in one month, and you believe you should get an additional 4 percent increase based on your excellent performance. What should your hourly wage be next week, and what do you anticipate it will be after your performance evaluation?

8. Last year, you purchased equipment in the HIM department for $10,250. You have been told that the equipment you bought has depreciated in value by 15 percent. What is the value of the equipment now?

9. You just scored 15 correct out of a possible 40 on your health information test. What percentage did you earn?

10. Last year, the number of hospitals in your state decreased from 320 to 240. What is the percentage of decrease?

11. During the last week Community Hospital reported that the following number of patients were discharged:

    Sunday—18; Monday—22; Tuesday—37; Wednesday—25; Thursday—22; Friday—28; Saturday—12.

    What is the average number of patients discharged during the week? (Round to a whole number.)

For the following questions, refer to the Quarterly Coder Accuracy Report on the next page.

12. Are the calculations of the percentage of records accurately coded for each month and the total for the quarter correct?

13. Coder D determined her accuracy rate for the quarter to be 95.1 percent. She would like you to recalculate her accuracy rate because she thinks it is incorrect.

Chapter 2 Test (continued)

Community Hospital
Quarterly Coder Accuracy Report
January–March 20XX

	January			February			March			Totals		
	# Records	# Correct	% Correct	# Records	# Correct	% Correct	# Records	# Correct	% Correct	# Records	# Correct	% Correct
Coder A	560	504	90.0%	544	495	91.0%	270	243	90.0%	1374	1242	90.4%
Coder B	540	503	93.1%	523	491	93.9%	531	494	93.0%	1594	1488	93.4%
Coder C	500	440	88.0%	445	401	90.1%	493	435	88.2%	1438	1276	88.7%
Coder D	620	583	94.0%	588	570	96.9%	584	551	94.3%	1792	1704	95.1%
Coder E	480	408	85.0%	432	392	90.7%	465	397	85.4%	1377	1197	86.9%
Total	**2700**	**2438**	**90.3%**	**2532**	**2349**	**92.8%**	**2343**	**2120**	**90.5%**	**7575**	**6907**	**91.2%**

Chapter 3
Patient Census Data

Objectives

At the conclusion of this chapter, you should be able to:

- Define, differentiate, and apply the terms inpatient census, daily inpatient census, inpatient service day, total inpatient service days, and admission and discharge (A&D)

- Differentiate between an interhospital (interfacility) transfer and an intrahospital transfer

- Compute daily census and inpatient service days using the admission and discharge data provided

- Compute census and inpatient service days with data given for births and transfers

- Compute the average daily census for a patient care unit given inpatient service days for any such unit

Inpatient Census

Hospital management uses census data for various purposes, including planning, budgeting, and staffing. The **inpatient census** indicates the number of patients present in the healthcare facility at a particular point in time. Hospitals only include inpatients in their calculations.

An individual on each **patient care unit** (PCU) is designated to count the patients on that unit each day. The inpatient census-taking time is usually at midnight (12:00 a.m.) but may occur at any time as long as the time is consistent for the entire facility, that is, each PCU conducts the census at the same time. Around midnight is actually a good time to take the census because patients are usually in their beds. It would be difficult to account for all patients at 8:00 a.m., for example, because they might not be in their beds. They may be in exam rooms, radiology, surgery, with their healthcare provider, or just taking a walk in the hospital.

In a manual system, the census taker fills out a form to be sent to a central collection area (usually the nursing office, information systems, admissions, health information department, or any other office designated by the administration). The names of patients admitted, discharged, and transferred to or from a PCU appear on the form. This makes it easier for the central collection area to discover any discrepancies in the data from the PCUs and to know where each patient is located at all times.

In a computerized system, the necessary data are first entered into the computer as admissions, discharges, or transfers and then verified at the designated time by the responsible person on each PCU.

> **Handy Tip:** A PCU is an organizational entity of a healthcare facility such as a medicine unit, surgery unit, or special unit such as the intensive care unit (ICU) or cardiac care unit (CCU). This should not be confused with medical services, which refer to the activities relating to medical care performed by physicians, nurses, and other healthcare professionals and technical personnel under the direction of a physician.

Table 3.1 shows a form for a manual daily census summary for a nursing home.

Complete Master Census

In addition to reporting the head count to the central collection area, each PCU reports, in written form or via computer, the number of patients admitted, discharged, and/or transferred in or out that day. This is commonly referred to as the ADT system in a facility. The central collection area then uses the census from all the units to compile a total census for the hospital, sometimes referred to as the **complete master census**. The complete master census shows the names of patients present in the hospital at a particular point in time and their location. In most facilities this is a computerized process that is linked with the facility's master patient index, billing system, and other electronic health record systems.

> **Handy Tip:** In this book, the term *transfer* in a hospital setting refers to an intrahospital transfer. **Intrahospital transfers** are patients who are moved from one PCU to another within the facility. The transfers in and transfers out on an individual PCU may not be equal because it is possible to transfer more patients in than transfer out and vice versa. However, the total intrahospital transfers in must always equal the intrahospital transfers out.

Table 3.1.   Daily Census Summary at Community Manor Nursing Home

To be completed daily at 12:01 a.m. by charge nurse			Community Manor Nursing Home Daily Census Summary	
Hall: ____A ____B ____C ____D			**Date** _____	
Initial admits—New residents			Date	Time
				a.m.–p.m.
				a.m.–p.m.
				a.m.–p.m.
				a.m.–p.m.
Discharged to home or transfer			Date	Time
				a.m.–p.m.
				a.m.–p.m.
				a.m.–p.m.
Transfer to hospital	Location		Date	Time
				a.m.–p.m.
				a.m.–p.m.
				a.m.–p.m.
				a.m.–p.m.
Out on leave—Pass	Date Left	Time	Returned	Time
		a.m.–p.m.		a.m.–p.m.
		a.m.–p.m.		a.m.–p.m.
		a.m.–p.m.		a.m.–p.m.
Deceased			Date	Time of Death
				a.m.–p.m.
				a.m.–p.m.
				a.m.–p.m.
Return from hospital stay			Date	Time
				a.m.–p.m.
				a.m.–p.m.
				a.m.–p.m.
				a.m.–p.m.

Charge nurse: _____

Exercise 3.1

Answer the following questions.

1. Unit A has a count of 20 patients at 1 a.m. on September 1 and 30 patients at the same time on September 2. Could the counts have been different if unit A had taken a census at 12:01 a.m. on both days?

2. Would you accept the different PCUs in the hospital taking censuses at different times as long as each unit is consistent within itself?

3. A patient transferred at 5 p.m. to unit A from unit B is counted in unit A's 12:01 a.m. census as one additional patient present. Would that patient still be included in unit B's 12:01 a.m. census?

Daily Inpatient Census

The **daily inpatient census** includes the number of inpatients present on the PCU at the census-taking time each day *and* any inpatients who were both admitted after the previous census-taking time and discharged before the next census-taking time. Thus, a patient admitted to the PCU at 8 a.m. on June 1 and discharged at 10 p.m. that same day would not be present for the PCU's head count. Therefore, he or she would not appear on the census report. However, the patient must be accounted for separately in some manner. For example, 20 patients are on the PCU. One patient was admitted at 10:00 a.m. and discharged at 7:00 p.m. If there are no discharges, the daily inpatient census for this day is 21. You add the patient who was admitted and discharged to the 20 patients already on the unit.

Exercise 3.2

Answer the following questions.

1. The census at 12:01 a.m. on June 1 is 107. Two patients are admitted on June 1 at 6:00 a.m. and discharged at 7:00 p.m. that same day. One patient admitted at 3:00 p.m. died at 5:30 p.m. the same afternoon. What is the PCU's daily census for June 1?

2. Which would be the better form of data to keep permanently, census or daily inpatient census? Why?

3. Community Hospital's census at 12:01 a.m. on September 16 was 256. On that day, 18 patients were admitted and 22 patients were discharged. Calculate the census for September 16.

4. Community Hospital's ICU census at 12:01 a.m. on December 2 was 19. Four patients were admitted to the ICU on December 2, one was discharged to the medicine unit, and two patients died. Calculate the census for the ICU for December 2.

Inpatient Service Days

An **inpatient service day** is a unit of measure denoting the services received by one inpatient in one 24-hour period. The 24-hour period is the time between the census-taking hours on two successive days. The usual 24-hour reporting period begins at 12:01 a.m. and ends at 12:00 p.m. (midnight). One inpatient service day is counted for each **inpatient admission** when a patient is admitted and discharged on the same day. If this is not done, credit for the services given to that patient is lost.

There are a number of important issues concerning inpatient service days. These include:

- One unit of one service day is not usually divided or reported as a fraction of a day.

- The day of admission is counted as an inpatient service day, but the day of discharge is not.

- The days a patient does not occupy a bed due to **leave of absence** are excluded because he or she is not present at the census-taking hour. A leave of absence day is a day occurring after the admission and prior to the discharge of a hospital inpatient when the patient is not present at the census-taking hour because he or she is on leave of absence from the healthcare facility. An absence of less than one day is not considered a leave of absence in compiling statistics. A leave of absence is not common in short-term acute care hospitals because lengths of stay are usually short. However, long-term care facilities such as nursing homes, mental health, drug and alcohol abuse and rehabilitation, or facilities for the developmentally disabled may still use them for special reasons such as a special holiday or outing for the patient or a group of patients, a family wedding, a funeral, or if the physician is trying to determine how well a patient would fare outside the facility. Leave of absence days are always written as a physician order. When the patient or the physician believes the advantages of an absence from the facility outweigh the advantages of uninterrupted **hospitalization**, the hospital has the choice of discharging and then readmitting the patient or granting a leave of absence.

*Inpatient service d*ay is the correct term to use for what is commonly referred to as a **patient day**, inpatient day, bed occupancy day, or **census day**. The operative word here is service, that is, the number of patients who received service on a particular day. The correct wording reflects the hospital function of providing services to patients each day. If 20 patients are provided services in one 24-hour period, the number of inpatient service days for that calendar day is 20.

Exercise 3.3

Compare the definition of inpatient service day to the definitions of inpatient daily census and census. Will the figure representing an inpatient service day for any one day be the same as the figure for a daily census or census?

Total Inpatient Service Days

The term **total inpatient service days** refers to the sum of all the inpatient service days in a period under consideration. For example, if the inpatient service days for June 1, 2, and 3 are 100, 105, and 101, the total for the three days is 306. Typically, total inpatient service days are calculated monthly, quarterly, semiannually, or annually.

Exercise 3.4

Given the following inpatient service days for a 65-bed hospital, what is the total number of inpatient service days provided in June?

Date June	Inpatient Service Days	Date June	Inpatient Service Days	Date June	Inpatient Service Days
1	62	11	58	21	63
2	62	12	57	22	59
3	63	13	55	23	52
4	61	14	52	24	56
5	59	15	51	25	54
6	58	16	49	26	58
7	60	17	54	27	53
8	61	18	56	28	54
9	64	19	58	29	59
10	59	20	59	30	63

Exercise 3.5

Complete the following exercises.

1. The difference between the census and the inpatient daily census is that any patients admitted and discharged the same day are added to:

   a. The census to compute the daily census
   b. The 12:01 a.m. (or other designated time) head count to compute the daily census
   c. Both a and b
   d. None of the above

Exercise 3.5 (continued)

2. Which of the following should be used when calculating the number of inpatients who received service on a particular day?

   a. The census
   b. The daily census
   c. Total inpatient service days
   d. None of the above

3. The time for taking the inpatient census must always be:

   a. Midnight
   b. Consistent
   c. 12:00 p.m.
   d. 11:59 a.m.

4. At census-taking time, a patient who has been transferred into a unit is:

   a. Counted where he or she is
   b. Counted where he or she came from
   c. Not counted
   d. Counted in both units

5. Patient day or inpatient day is more correctly termed:

   a. Inpatient service day
   b. Daily inpatient census
   c. Total inpatient service day(s)
   d. Census

6. The inpatient census at 12:01 a.m. is 57. Two patients were admitted at 1 p.m. and one died at 3:15 p.m. and the other was discharged at 10:00 p.m. The inpatient service days for that day are:

   a. 50
   b. 55
   c. 57
   d. 59

7. Define the following terms:

   a. Census
   b. Daily inpatient census
   c. Inpatient service day
   d. Total inpatient service days

Calculation of Inpatient Service Days

The **calculation of inpatient service days** is the measurement of services received by all inpatients in one 24-hour period (the time between the census-taking hours on two successive days). The usual reporting period begins at 12:01 a.m. and ends at 12:00 p.m.

(midnight). Moreover, one inpatient day must be counted for each inpatient admitted and discharged on the same day between two successive census-taking hours.

> **Example:** The definitions of census, inpatient service day, and total inpatient service days provide clues for actual computation. The sample shown in table 3.2 includes all of a hospital's inpatient care units. A summary of all such units helps the administration review the hospital's overall level of activity.
>
> **Handy Tip:** Sometimes you may be asked by the administration to exclude PCUs such as intensive care units (ICUs) and obstetrical units from the inpatient service days. Units such as these are studied separately because the intensity of service on these units varies greatly from the intensity of services provided on medical/surgical units. Moreover, hospital administration may want information regarding usage on these units in order to determine equipment and staffing needs. Hospitals may use inpatient service days to track trends from month-to-month or year-to-date.

Table 3.3 shows a sample of how hospital administration can use inpatient service days data to determine performance.

Table 3.2.   Sample Inpatient Service Days Display

Sample Inpatient Services Days	
Number of patients in hospital at 12:01 a.m. on November 1	467
Plus the number of patients admitted on November 1	+ 54
Subtotal	521
Minus the number of patients discharged (including deaths) on November 1	− 45
Number of patients in hospital at 11:59 p.m. on November 1 (subtotal)	476
Plus the number of patients both admitted and discharged on November 1	+ 3
Total inpatient service days for November 1	479

Table 3.3.   Year-to-Date Inpatient Service Days

Community Medical Center September, 20XX Year-to-Date Inpatient Service Days			
Service	**Actual**	**Budget**	**Prior Year**
Medicine	12,652	15,000	14,097
Surgery	9,853	13,500	12,440
Intensive Care	2,652	3,500	2,750
Step-down	987	1,500	1,300
Rehabilitation	1,522	2,500	2,000
Obstetrics	1,621	2,200	2,160
Psychiatry	988	1,000	1,204
Newborn	1,356	1,800	1,458
Neonatal ICU	2,965	3,900	2,812
Pediatrics	528	1,000	1,523
Total	**35,124**	**45,900**	**41,744**

This medical center's analysis of its inpatient service days can be examined to determine how well the facility is doing year-to-date and compare its performance to the previous year. This can lead to discussions by administration concerning marketing of their services or examination whether there are enough practitioners in those services that may not be doing as well as in the previous year.

Before beginning the actual calculation of census data and inpatient service days, it is important to understand the term **calculation of transfers**. The calculation of transfers occurs on the PCU census. Transfers in and out of the unit are shown as subdivisions of patients admitted to and discharged from the unit.

Example: Following are some sample figures listed in a format frequently used by the central collection area: A head count at 12:01 a.m. on June 1 shows 48 adult and children inpatients and two newborns. Using this starting point, add the number of admissions (2) and transfers in (1) to the number of adult and children inpatients (48) to arrive at a total of 51.

Note: Below, a/d indicates admitted and discharged the same day; adm, admissions; b, births; dis, discharges; inpt, inpatients; Nb, newborns; A/C, adults and children; serv, service; and trf, transfer.

↓   +   +   ↓

Day	12:01 a.m. census A/C	Nb	adm A/C	b	trf in	total A/C	Nb	dis A/C	dis Nb	trf out	11:59 p.m. census A/C	Nb	a/d	serv days A/C	Nb
6/1	**48**	2	**2**	1	**1**	51	3	1	2	1	49	1	1	50	1

Add the births (1) to the newborns present at 12:01 a.m. to arrive at a total of three.

↓   +   ↓

Day	12:01 a.m. census A/C	Nb	adm A/C	b	trf in	total A/C	Nb	dis A/C	dis Nb	trf out	11:59 p.m. census A/C	Nb	a/d	serv days A/C	Nb
6/1	48	**2**	2	**1**	1	51	**3**	1	2	1	49	1	1	50	1

Subtract the discharges A/C (1) and the transfers out A/C (1) to the number of adults and children (51) for an 11:59 p.m. census of 49.

↓   −   −   ↓

Day	12:01 a.m. census A/C	Nb	adm A/C	b	trf in	total A/C	Nb	dis A/C	dis Nb	trf out	11:59 p.m. census A/C	Nb	a/d	serv days A/C	Nb
6/1	48	2	2	1	1	**51**	3	**1**	2	**1**	**49**	1	1	50	1

Finally, subtract the newborns that were discharged (2) from the total number of newborns (3) for an 11:59 p.m. census of one.

↓   −   ↓

Day	12:01 a.m. census A/C	Nb	adm A/C	b	trf in	total A/C	Nb	dis A/C	dis Nb	trf out	11:59 p.m. census A/C	Nb	a/d	serv days A/C	Nb
6/1	48	2	2	1	1	51	**3**	1	**2**	1	49	**1**	1	50	1

The last two columns are discussed later in this chapter.

The following points should resolve any confusion:

- The terms *transfers in* and *transfers out* refer to intrahospital transfers, that is, transfers within the hospital. Transfers in and out of the hospital (called interhospital or interfacility transfers) are included in admissions and discharges. It is common for healthcare providers to use the term *transfer,* as in "The patient was transferred to the nursing home." However, this is really a discharge from the hospital and an admission to the nursing home.

- Transfers in and out of any specific medical care unit may or may not be equal, but they must be equal for the overall hospital **recapitulation.** Every patient transferred into a unit on any given day has to have been transferred out of another unit. Failure of these data to balance may mean that a unit neglected to report transfers correctly. It is essential that someone in the central collection area identify the source of error.

- The data of 49 adults and children and one newborn (the inpatient census at 11:59 p.m. on June 1) must be the same as the actual head count. If they are not the same, a unit may have reported admissions, discharges, or births incorrectly. Again, someone in the central collection area is responsible for finding the error.

- Newborns are considered separately for all computations based on census data. They should be reported separately unless otherwise directed by administration, medical staff, or other persons using the statistical data produced. Births are considered newborn admissions. As mentioned earlier, services provided to newborns differ in intensity from those provided to the rest of the hospital inpatients.

- The census at the close of one day (11:59 p.m.) is the inpatient census at the beginning of the next day and is commonly referred to as the number of patients remaining. This may be a good time to discuss the terminology used in inpatient settings. The hospital may be referred to as the "house", as in "How many patients are in the house?" This refers to the number of patients in the hospital.

Patients Admitted and Discharged on the Same Day

Going back to the last two columns from the previous problem on p. 31, the number of patients who were admitted and discharged on the same day (a/d) must be added to the 11:59 p.m. census to show that they received services. These are the inpatient service days. As discussed previously, patients who are not present at either of two successive head-counting times still must be accounted for and credited with a day's care. (A patient admitted and discharged on the same day may be referred to as in and out [I&O] or admission/discharge [A&D] or any number of other terms or abbreviations.)

To compute inpatient service days, add the number of patients admitted and discharged on the same day (a/d) to the 11:59 p.m. census data. Note the 50 and 1 in the last column for June 1.

> **Handy Tip:** The census for the next day must begin with the 11:59 p.m. census data and not inpatient service days. Calculate under the assumption that the patients admitted and discharged on the same day and the transfers are not newborns.

Recapitulation of Census Data

The process of verifying the data obtained by the process described above is called the monthly or yearly recapitulation of census data, meaning a summary of the data. The total number of patients admitted and born during the month or year is added to the patients-remaining census with which the month or year began. From this sum, the number of discharges (including deaths) during the month or year is subtracted. The resulting data are the number of patients remaining at the end of the month or year. This number should equal the actual head count at 11:59 p.m. the last night of that month or year. Table 3.4 shows a sample monthly census recapitulation.

When you recap (or summarize) monthly (or annual) census data, you are verifying that the columns have been added correctly. This procedure also verifies that no error was made in the original data on one or more lines. This is accomplished by taking the 12:01 a.m. inpatient census at the beginning of the period, adding total admissions and transfers in, and subtracting total discharges and transfers out. The resultant data represent the ending census on the last day of the period (month or year).

Table 3.4.　Sample Monthly Census Recapitulation

Community Hospital		
	Adults and Children	**Newborns**
Number of patients in hospital at 12:01 a.m. on October 1	48	2
Add the number of patients admitted in October	+ 100	+ 7
Subtotal	148	9
Subtract the number of patients discharged (including deaths) in October	− 110	− 5
Number of patients in hospital at 11:59 p.m., October 31	38	4

Exercise 3.6

Complete the following exercises.

1. Using the data given on page 31, calculate the census for June 2. Then fill in the blanks in the table below. Did the transfers in and transfers out balance?

	12:01 a.m. census		adm		trf	total		dis	dis	trf	11:59 p.m. census			serv days	
Day	A/C	Nb	A/C	b	in	A/C	Nb	A/C	Nb	out	A/C	Nb	a/d	A/C	Nb
6/1	48	2	2	1	1	51	3	1	2	1	49	1			
6/2			3	1	2			4	1	2					

(continued on next page)

Exercise 3.6 (continued)

2. What data will you use to begin June 3, and why?

3. Fill in the blanks in the table below. What are the inpatient service days for June 2 and 3?

	12:01 a.m. census		adm		trf	total		dis	dis	trf	11:59 p.m. census			serv days	
Day	A/C	Nb	A/C	b	in	A/C	Nb	A/C	Nb	out	A/C	Nb	a/d	A/C	Nb
6/1	48	2	2	1	1	51	3	1	2	1	49	1	1	50	1
6/2	49	1	3	1	2	54	2	4	1	2	48	1	1		
6/3			1	1	1			3	0	1			0		

4. Would a newborn ever be considered an a/d?

5. At this point, you have inpatient service days for three successive days. The total of these data, excluding newborns, for June 1, 2, and 3 is 145 (50 + 49 + 46). What will you need to know and do to get the hospital total inpatient service days for the entire month of June?

Exercise 3.7

Using the information supplied for June 1, fill in the blanks in the table below.

	12:01 am. census		adm		trf	total		dis	dis	trf	11:59 p.m. census			serv days	
Day	A/C	Nb	A/C	b	in	A/C	Nb	A/C	Nb	out	A/C	Nb	a/d	A/C	Nb
6/1	250	18	20	4	2			25	3	2			1		
6/2			22	6	1			24	5	1			0		
6/3			24	5	0			23	4	0			3		
6/4			22	3	1			22	3	1			1		
6/5			25	4	2			25	3	2			2		

Exercise 3.8

Two hundred adults and children were in the hospital at 12:01 a.m. on August 1. There were 42 newborns at 12:01 a.m. on August 1. During August, the following data are compiled:

Admissions:

Adults and children	1,567
Newborns	97

Discharges (including deaths):

Adults and children	1,572
Newborns	107

1. What would the inpatient census for adults and children be on August 31 at 11:59 p.m.?

2. What would the inpatient census be for newborns on August 31?

3. Can the inpatient service days be computed with the information supplied in the previous question? Explain why or why not.

4. The surgery unit in Community Hospital has reported the following data. Do these data look correct? Explain.

Day	12:01 a.m. census	Adm	Trf In	Total	Disch	Trf Out	11:59 p.m. census	A/D	Serv Days
6/1	50	6	3	59	9	1	49	1	50

Exercise 3.9

This exercise consists of two worksheets for calculating a month's inpatient census and inpatient service days. Using the data provided for May 1, complete the first worksheet. If your findings do not match the data for May 31, you have made an error either in your column additions or on one or more of the horizontal lines above the total. You must correct this error to ensure the validity of the monthly totals. If the column additions are correct, continue on to the second worksheet for the recap. This exercise could be placed on an electronic spreadsheet.

Worksheet No. 1

Day	12:01 a.m. census A/C	NB	Adm A/C	bir	Trf in	Total A/C	NB	Disch A/C	NB	Trf out	11:59 p.m. census A/C	NB	A/D	Serv days A/C	NB
1	162	2	22	1	10	194	3	19	0	10	165	3	1	166	3
2	165	3	29	0	8			23	1	8			0		
3			14	2	3			24	0	3			1		
4			24	0	5			25	0	5			0		
5			11	1	6			25	2	6			0		
6			20	0	1			16	0	1			0		
7			29	0	10			17	0	10			0		
8			24	2	13			20	0	13			3		
9			23	1	7			22	1	7			1		
10			19	0	10			17	0	10			0		
11			11	0	5			22	3	5			1		
12			16	0	6			24	0	6			0		
13			18	1	5			25	0	5			0		
14			29	0	5			19	0	5			0		
15			28	0	8			22	2	8			1		
16			26	3	6			19	0	6			0		
17			26	0	7			19	2	7			0		
18			18	0	10			25	0	10			0		
19			12	0	6			33	0	6			0		
20			22	1	8			16	3	8			1		
21			26	0	3			17	0	3			1		
22			32	2	11			25	0	11			1		
23			29	2	14			27	0	14			0		
24			22	0	10			21	2	10			0		
25			20	3	13			34	0	13			0		

Exercise 3.9 (continued)

26			14	0	6			37	1	6			1		
27			23	0	5			16	0	5			0		
28			26	2	4			18	2	4			0		
29			17	0	6			22	1	6			1		
30			19	0	7			21	1	7			0		
31			21	1	12			16	0	12	146	3	1	147	3

Worksheet No. 2

Recap of Monthly Data for Adults and Children: May 20XX
(Enter numbers from Worksheet #1)

12:01 a.m. Census A/C   162

Adm A/C   + _____

Trf In   + _____

Total A/C   = _____

Disch A/C   − _____

Trf Out   − _____

11:59 p.m. Census A/C   =   146

Recap of Monthly Data for Newborns:

12:01 a.m. Census NB   2

Bir   + _____

Total NB   = _____

Disch NB   − _____

11:59 p.m. Census NB   =   3

Serv Days A/C (total inpatient service days excluding newborns) _____

Serv days NB (total newborn service days) _____

Total inpatient service days _____

Average Daily Inpatient Census

The **average daily census** is the average number of inpatients present each day for a given period of time. The total inpatient service days for any period (usually a month or a year) represents the inpatient service days for all the calendar days in that period. The formula for calculating average daily census is:

$$\frac{Total\ inpatient\ service\ days\ for\ a\ period\ (excluding\ newborns)}{Total\ number\ of\ days\ in\ the\ period}$$

When calculating the average daily census for a month, you need to know how many days there are in each month. Remember the nursery rhyme?

> *Thirty days hath September, April, June, and November.*
> *All the rest have thirty-one.*
> *Excepting February alone,*
> *Which has twenty-eight days clear,*
> *But twenty-nine each Leap Year.*

Example: In the second worksheet in exercise 3.9 starting on page 36, the answer was 4,868 inpatient service days for adults and children and 91 inpatient service days for newborns for the month of May. According to the formula, the average daily census is computed by dividing 4,868 by 31 (number of days in May). The result is 157.03, or, rounded to a whole number, 157.

Handy Tip: Because patient load can fluctuate, the administration is very interested in the hospital's average daily inpatient census. For example, many healthcare facilities in the South experience a rise in average daily census during the winter months and a decrease during the summer months due to seasonal visitors. The average daily inpatient census is a measure of use and a reference for anticipated revenues.

As mentioned earlier, adults and children are calculated separately from newborns unless otherwise directed by the hospital's administration. Newborn census data can distort statistics related to resource use. For example, it costs less to maintain a newborn nursery than it does to staff other PCUs. If the average daily census is consistently low over a specified period, it may be appropriate to close PCUs to reduce expenses. In this example, the average daily newborn census is calculated by dividing 91 by 31. The result is 2.94 or 3.

Handy Tip: Whether or not to round to a whole number is the individual hospital's decision. What is important is that the hospital act consistently. There is a difference between working with data representing people (because you cannot have a portion of a person) and working with percentages that represent numbers. Many facilities use a whole number when calculating the census and fractions with other healthcare statistics. (See chapter 2 for a discussion of rounding.)

Example: A 100-bed hospital reports 2,579 inpatient service days for October. To compute the average daily inpatient census for October, divide 2,579 by 31 (number of days in October). The average daily inpatient census is 83.19 or when rounded to a whole number is 83. This simply means that on average, 83 patients were in the facility during each day in October.

Again, this number is very important to administration because they will want to know how many patients are being served each month in order to determine staffing and supply needs for practitioners and to monitor the overall financial performance of the facility.

Average Daily Newborn Census

The formula for calculating the average daily census for newborns follows the same pattern as the formula for calculating the average daily census of adults and children.

$$\frac{Total\ newborn\ inpatient\ service\ days\ for\ a\ period}{Total\ number\ of\ days\ in\ the\ period}$$

Example: A hospital with 25 bassinets had 652 newborn inpatient service days during September. Divide the total number of newborn inpatient service days (652) by the number of days in the period (30 days in September) to obtain the average daily newborn census (21.7333, or 22).

Handy Tip: When administrators and physicians ask for the average daily inpatient census, they may not always indicate to exclude newborns. Clarify the information by asking if newborns should be included or excluded from your computations.

Average Daily Census for a Patient Care Unit

The hospital's administration often finds it helpful to know the average use of a specific medical care unit (for example, to know whether additional beds are needed for the ICU). Statistics are the basis for decision making. The formula for calculating the average daily census for a care unit is:

$$\frac{Total\ inpatient\ service\ days\ for\ the\ unit\ for\ the\ period}{Total\ number\ of\ days\ in\ the\ period}$$

Example: A hospital with a 15-bed cardiac care unit reports 450 inpatient service days for July. To compute the average daily census, divide 450 by 31 (number of days in July). The average daily census is 14.5 or 15. This indicates that the cardiac care unit is, on average, filled to capacity each day. Administration may want to consider this information closely to determine if additional beds may be needed.

Handy Tip: Some of the exercises in this textbook cover leap years. A leap year is a year in which an extra day is added to the calendar in order to harmonize with the seasons. It takes the Earth 365.2422 days to complete its course around the Sun; thus, a leap year must be added roughly once every four years. The extra day in a leap year is called a leap day and is added to the end of February, giving February 29 days.

Exercise 3.10

Complete the following exercises.

1. Community Hospital has 200 beds and 25 newborn bassinets. The total inpatient service days for February, in a non-leap year, were 4,879 for adults and children and 658 for newborns. What is the average daily census (rounded to a whole number)?

2. A 150-bed, 15-bassinet hospital has 3,264 inpatient service days for adults and children and 365 newborn service days during November. What is the average daily census, excluding newborns? Round to a whole number.

3. Compute the average daily newborn census for a 100-bed, 10-bassinet hospital with 2,589 inpatient service days for adults and children and 257 inpatient service days for newborns during September. Round your answer to a whole number.

4. If you need to calculate the average daily census of the Surgical unit, where can you obtain the Surgical unit's inpatient service days?

5. Community Hospital's Burn unit has 7 beds. The inpatient service days for January were 199. What is the average daily census for the Burn unit during January? Round your answer to a whole number.

6. Community Hospital reports the following:

Community Hospital
December, 20XX

	Adults and children	Nursery
Beginning Census on December 1	86	8
Admissions	248	62
Discharges and deaths	217	59
Inpatient service days	2,022	248

   a. Calculate the average daily inpatient census for adults and children.
   b. Calculate the average daily inpatient census for the nursery.
   c. What will the census for adults and children be at 11:59 p.m. on December 31?
   d. What will the newborn census be at 11:59 p.m. on December 31?

7. Go back to the information given in No. 1 and determine the newborn average daily census. Round to a whole number.

8. Go back to the information given in No. 2 and determine the newborn average daily census. Round to a whole number.

Chapter 3 Test

1. Differentiate between the terms *census* and *daily inpatient census*.

2. What is an intrahospital transfer?

3. Is it possible that the transfers into a patient care unit may not equal the transfers out of the same patient care unit on the same day?

4. When must transfers in and transfer out be equal?

5. At 11:59 p.m. on January 1, Community Hospital census was 321. On January 2, 73 patients were admitted, 24 were discharged and 3 were admitted and died that day. On their ICU unit the census on January 1 was 12. On January 2, 4 patients were admitted, 3 were discharged, and 1 was admitted and later that day died in the ICU. Answer the following questions and round the answers to whole numbers.

   a. Calculate the inpatient census for January 2.
   b. Calculate the hospital daily inpatient census for January 2.
   c. Calculate the ICU inpatient service days for January 2.

6. In 20XX, a hospital had 150 beds for adults and children from January 1 through June 30. On July 1, the hospital increased its beds to 200 and the number remained at 200 through December 31. During the first six months, 27,813 patient days of service were provided to the hospital's adults and children. During the last six months, 35,873 days of service were provided. Answer the following questions and round the answers to whole numbers. This is non-leap year.

   a. What was the average daily census for the first six months: 153, 154, 155, or 156?
   b. What was the average daily census for the entire year: 173, 174, 175, or 193?
   c. The same hospital provided 7,890 newborn days of service in its 30-bassinet nursery during the year. What was the average daily newborn census: 20, 21, 22, or 23?
   d. The same hospital's surgery unit has 45 beds. During July, the unit provided 2,002 days of service. What was the average daily census for the surgery unit in July: 28: 60, 62, 63, or 65?

(continued on next page)

Chapter 3 Test (continued)

7. Using the statistics from the following monthly report from the nursing administration of Community Hospital, an acute care facility, calculate the current month's (June) average daily census for each nursing unit and the totals. Note that this facility's policy is to round to a whole number.

Community Hospital
Inpatient Statistical Report
Average Daily Census by Nursing Unit
June, 20XX

	Unit	Inpatient Service Days	Average Daily Census
A	Obstetrical	520	
B	Pediatric	87	
C	Medicine/Surgery	6,176	
D	Medicine ICU	383	
E	Surgery ICU	307	
F	Psychiatry	603	
G	Rehabilitation	725	
H	Cardiac Care Unit	213	
Total Adult and Children		9,014	
I	Newborn Nursery	475	
J	Special Care Nursery	135	
K	Neonatal ICU	408	
Total Nursery		1,018	

Chapter 4
Percentage of Occupancy

Objectives

At the conclusion of this chapter, you should be able to:

- Define and differentiate among the terms inpatient bed count, bed complement, total bed count days, newborn bassinet count, bed count days, newborn bassinet count days

- Identify the beds that are included in a bed count

- Compute the bed occupancy percentage for any period given the data representing bed count and inpatient service days (adults and children)

- Compute the bassinet occupancy percentage for any period given bassinet count and newborn inpatient service days (newborn)

- Compute the percentage of occupancy for a period when there has been a change in the number of beds during that period

- Calculate the direct and indirect bed turnover rate

Inpatient Bed Count

Typically, a healthcare facility is licensed by the state to operate with a specific number of beds. When a new facility wants to open its doors for patient care, or when an existing hospital wants to add services or major medical equipment, it may need to apply to the state for a **certificate of need** (CON) to prove that patient care beds are needed in the area. Certificate of need programs are designed to contain healthcare facility costs and prevent the duplication of services and construction. Thirty-six states require a CON program. When granted a CON, the facility is licensed for the specific number of beds requested and is responsible for reporting its bed count.

A **bed count**, also called an **inpatient bed count**, is the number of available **hospital inpatient beds**, both occupied and vacant, on any given day. In a hospital, the bed count includes those beds set up for normal use, whether or not they are occupied. A bed count may be reported for the entire hospital or for any of its units. Normally, when counting inpatient beds, only those in areas designed for such accommodations and set up, staffed, equipped, and in all respects ready for the care of inpatients are counted. This is an important consideration because regulatory agency surveyors often verify bed count and location against licensed beds and appropriate staffing levels. The bed count may be used in various reports, from those prepared for accrediting agencies to those prepared for regulatory agencies. In a hospital, the number of available beds in the facility or a unit may remain constant for long periods of time. At times, however, the number can change. For example, a significant number of beds may be unavailable for use during a major remodeling or renovation project, but the number will increase after the project is completed. Another example is during a disaster, natural or otherwise. Regular beds may be occupied so additional beds would be set up in alcoves or hallways or other areas that are not considered patient rooms. These beds do not become a part of the regular bed count. Some facilities refer to these as disaster beds. Therefore, it is imperative to do a bed count.

Bed complement is an alternate term for bed count, and bed capacity sometimes is used synonymously with bed count and bed complement (although its use has led to some confusion). Bed capacity also can denote the number of beds that a facility has been designed and constructed to contain, rather than the actual number of beds set up and staffed for use. To avoid confusion, it is preferable to use bed count.

Certain types of beds are excluded from the bed count, for example, those in treatment areas such as examining rooms, emergency services, physical therapy, labor rooms, and recovery rooms.

Labor Room Beds and Newborn Beds

An obstetrics patient may be admitted directly to a labor room bed instead of to a postpartum bed where she may spend the majority of her hospital stay. Labor room beds are not included in the bed count because they are used only temporarily before the patient delivers.

Newborn beds called bassinets are computed separately from the bed count. The **newborn bassinet count** is the number of available **hospital newborn bassinets**, both occupied and vacant, on any given day.

Emergency Services Department Beds

Emergency services department (ESD) beds are normally considered outpatient beds. In some instances, however, the hospital provides an observation bed in the ESD. If observation beds meet the qualifications of being set up, equipped, and staffed for inpatient use, they may be counted in the bed count depending on what the particular facility has decided and on state-licensing compliance.

A patient under observation, an **observation patient**, needs to be monitored, evaluated, and assessed for admission to inpatient status or discharged for care to another setting. He or she can occupy a special bed set aside for this purpose or a bed in any unit of the hospital (that is, the ESD, a medical unit, or obstetrics). Usually hospital administration decides on the terms to describe and classify outpatients who occupy hospital beds and information systems to track these patients.

Exercise 4.1

In the event of a disaster, extra beds may be set up to meet the immediate needs of the situation. Would these beds be part of the bed count?

Bed Count Days

A **bed count day** is a unit of measure denoting the presence of one inpatient bed (either occupied or vacant) set up and staffed for use in one 24-hour period. The term **total bed count days** refers to the sum of inpatient bed count days for each of the days in the period under consideration. Bed count days also may be referred to as the maximum number of patient days or potential days because they represent a statistical probability of every bed being occupied every day.

> **Example:** A hospital has an inpatient bed count of 100. During September, the bed count days would be 100 (number of beds) × 30 (the number of days in September) or 3,000.

> If every hospital bed were filled each day for a certain period (for example, a month), the inpatient bed occupancy rate would be 100 percent for that month. This is because each bed was occupied the maximum number of times it could have been occupied.

> We can also use this for newborn bassinets. An inpatient bassinet count day is a unit of measure denoting the presence of one inpatient bassinet (either occupied or vacant) set up and staffed for use in one 24-hour period. The term total bassinet count days refers to the sum of inpatient bassinet count days for each of the days in the period under consideration.

> **Example:** A hospital has a bassinet count of 10. The bed count days in September would be 10 (number of bassinets) × 30 (the number of days in September) or 300.

All the rates in this text can be determined by remembering this general rule: A rate is the number of times something has happened compared to the number of times something could have happened. The equation is:

$$Rate = \frac{Part}{Base}$$

or:

$$\frac{The\ number\ of\ times\ something\ happened}{The\ number\ of\ times\ it\ could\ have\ happened}$$

The number of times "something happened" is expressed in terms of inpatient service days. The number of times "it could have happened" is expressed in terms of bed count days (bed count multiplied by the number of calendar days). (See chapter 2 for the discussion on rates.)

Bed Occupancy Ratio/Percentage

Occupancy percentages also are referred to as rates or ratios. The **bed occupancy ratio** is the proportion of beds occupied, defined as the ratio of inpatient service days to bed count days in the period under consideration. The inpatient service days are used to represent the actual occupancy (number of times something happened) and the bed count represents the possibility for occupancy (number of times it could have happened). The formula for determining bed occupancy ratio is:

$$\frac{Total\ inpatient\ service\ days\ in\ a\ period \times 100}{Total\ bed\ count\ days\ in\ the\ period\ (Bed\ count \times Number\ of\ days\ in\ the\ period)}$$

Synonymous terms for bed occupancy ratio are **percent of occupancy**, occupancy rate, **occupancy percent**, **percentage of occupancy**, and **occupancy ratio**. The ratio is usually expressed as a percent and can be computed for any specified day or as a daily average in any period of time.

Example: On June 1, 170 inpatient service days were provided in a 200-bed hospital. Making the appropriate substitutions in the previously stated formula, the bed occupancy ratio for June 1 is calculated as follows:

$$\frac{(170 \times 100)}{200} = \frac{17,000}{200} = 85\%$$

The bed occupancy ratio for June 1 is 85 percent. This simply means that on June 1, 85 percent of the beds were occupied.

Handy Tip: You might prefer to compute a decimal fraction and then multiply by 100. Another option is to convert to a percentage by moving the decimal point two places to the right as:

$$\frac{170}{200} = 0.85 = 85\%$$

Another example of bed occupancy ratio for the period of a month by patient care unit is shown in the following table.

Community Hospital
December 20XX

Patient Care Unit/ Bed Count	Inpatient Service Days	Percentage of Occupancy (Rounded to one decimal point)
Medicine/24 beds	731	$\dfrac{(731 \times 100)}{(24 \times 31)} = 98.25\% = 98.3\%$
Surgery/16 beds	392	$\dfrac{(392 \times 100)}{(16 \times 31)} = 79.0\%$
Rehabilitation/4 beds	97	$\dfrac{(97 \times 100)}{(4 \times 31)} = 78.2\%$
Obstetrics/6 beds	180	$\dfrac{(180 \times 100)}{(6 \times 31)} = 96.77\% = 96.8\%$
Total/50 beds	1,400	$\dfrac{(1400 \times 100)}{(50 \times 31)} = 90.3\%$

Example: The total bed occupancy ratio for December is 90.3 percent. Additionally, as the example shows, it is possible to compute the bed occupancy rate for individual patient care units (PCUs).

In another example, a hurricane hit a small coastal town on September 19, 20XX. The local hospital is licensed for 75 beds. All 75 beds were occupied; an additional 10 beds (disaster beds) were set up in the facility and occupied. The calculation for the percentage of occupancy for September 19 would be:

$$\frac{(85 \times 100)}{(75 \times 1)} = 113.3\%$$

This is an example of an instance where the percentage of occupancy is greater than 100 percent. This often happens in a disaster. Also important to note is that even though 10 additional beds were set up temporarily to handle the increased patient load, only the 75 beds are used in the denominator because they are the normal number of beds available. Remember that disaster beds or other beds set up for temporary use are not counted in the bed count.

Exercise 4.2

Using the information in the table below, calculate (round to one decimal place) the percentage of occupancy for each day of the month and for the entire month.

Community Hospital
September 20XX
75 beds

Date	Inpatient Service Days	Percentage of Occupancy	Date	Inpatient Service Days	Percentage of Occupancy
1	74		16	62	
2	73		17	61	
3	70		18	78	
4	71		19	75	
5	68		20	76	
6	67		21	77	
7	66		22	79	
8	54		23	72	
9	59		24	64	
10	69		25	58	
11	49		26	65	
12	52		27	63	
13	55		28	60	
14	56		29	53	
15	57		30	51	

Exercise 4.3

Using the information in the table below, calculate (round to one decimal place) the percentage of occupancy for each unit of Children's Hospital and the total (adults and children).

Children's Hospital
April, 20XX

Unit	Bed Count	Inpatient Service Days	Percentage of Occupancy
Pediatric Medicine	55	1,450	
Pediatric Surgery	40	1,059	
Respiratory	25	642	
Hematology/Oncology	38	1,122	
Pediatric ICU	12	275	
Pediatric Cardiac ICU	10	261	
Neonatal ICU	20	456	

Change in Bed Count

Occasionally, a hospital changes its bed count during a period of time. This expansion or reduction is a permanent change and is not designed to meet a temporary or emergency situation.

For example, a hospital changes its official bed count from 50 to 75 on January 15 and goes on to provide a total of 1,700 inpatient service days for the entire month. How is the maximum number of bed count days determined for the month of January? Multiply 50 beds by the first 14 days of the month and 75 beds by the remaining 17 days of the month, and then add the products.

$$14 \times 50 = 700$$

$$17 \times 75 = 1,275$$

$$700 + 1,275 = 1,975$$

The maximum number of bed count days for January is 1,975. Now compute the bed occupancy ratio. The calculation is:

$$\frac{(1,700 \times 100)}{1,975} = \frac{170,000}{1,975} = 86.07\% = 86.1\%$$

The bed occupancy ratio for January is 86.1 percent.

This procedure provides the most accurate result. Compare the previous computation with what would have happened if 50 beds had been used for the entire month. The calculation is:

$$\frac{(1,700 \times 100)}{(50 \times 31)} = \frac{17,000}{1,550} = 109.67 = 109.7\%$$

If 75 beds had been used for the entire month, the calculation would be:

$$\frac{(1,700 \times 100)}{(75 \times 31)} = \frac{170,000}{2,325} = 73.11 = 73.1\%$$

Obviously, there is a significant difference in the results. This example illustrates how easy it can be to present an inaccurate statistical picture. Because many administrative decisions are made on the basis of statistical presentations, the health information management (HIM) practitioner has an important responsibility in providing accurate data and validating computerized statistics.

Exercise 4.4

Community Hospital began the year 20XX, a non-leap year, with 102 beds. By March 1st, it had expanded the number of beds to 116. In April through June, the hospital reported 120 beds, which increased to 124 beds in July through October. Finally, the hospital completed its expansion process in November to end the year with 130 beds. Use these data to answer the questions below. Round to one decimal place.

Community Hospital
Annual Statistics, 20XX

Month	Bed Count (A/C)	Inpatient Service Days	Percentage of Occupancy
January	102	2,895	
February	102	2,796	
March	116	2,991	
April	120	3,078	
May	120	3,087	
June	120	3,396	
July	124	3,587	
August	124	3,656	
September	124	3,654	
October	124	3,698	
November	130	3,832	
December	130	3,765	

Exercise 4.4 (continued)

1. Calculate the percentage of occupancy for each month.

2. Calculate the percentage of occupancy for each quarter (January through March, April through June, July through September, and October through December).

3. Calculate the percentage of occupancy for the year.

Exercise 4.5

Using the statistics in the following report generated for Community Hospital, calculate (round to one decimal place) the percentage of occupancy for the month of December.

Community Hospital
December, 20XX

PCU	Inpatient Service Days	Bed Count	Percentage of Occupancy
Med/Surg	1,876	70	
ICU	300	10	
CCU	240	8	
Rehabilitation	300	12	
Burn	75	5	
Psychiatry	200	15	
Pediatric	870	30	
Total			
Nursery	280	10	

Newborn Bassinet Occupancy Ratio

Typically, newborn occupancy ratios are computed separately. If every bassinet were full every day in the period, the hospital would have the maximum potential bassinet occupancy. The formula for determining newborn bassinet occupancy is:

$$\frac{Total\ newborn\ inpatient\ service\ days\ for\ a\ period \times 100}{Total\ newborn\ bassinet\ count \times Number\ of\ days\ in\ the\ period}$$

Example: During March, a hospital with a bassinet count of 30 provided 810 newborn inpatient service days of care. According to the formula, the newborn bassinet occupancy ratio for March would be:

$$\frac{(810 \times 100)}{(30 \times 31)} = \frac{81,000}{930} = 87.09\% = 87.1\%$$

Exercise 4.6

Use the statistics in the following report generated for Community Hospital to make the following three calculations (non-leap year). Round to one decimal place.

Community Hospital
Annual Statistics 20XX

Newborn bassinets
January–March: 10
April–June: 12
July–September: 15
October–December: 20

Month	Newborn Inpatient Service Days	Percentage of Occupancy
January	300	
February	280	
March	307	
April	326	
May	355	
June	370	
July	427	
August	415	
September	430	
October	452	
November	444	
December	495	

1. Calculate the percentage of occupancy for each month.

2. Calculate the percentage of occupancy for each quarter (January through March, April through June, July through September, and October through December).

3. Calculate the percentage of occupancy for the year.

Bed Turnover Rate

The **bed turnover rate** refers to the number of times a bed, on average, changes occupants during a given period of time or the average number of admissions per bed per time period. The bed turnover rate is useful because two time periods may have the same percentage of occupancy, but the turnover rates may be different. For example, if a unit such as an obstetric unit has a high turnover rate, this could be an indication that the unit can accommodate more patients because the patients have a shorter length of stay (LOS). Conversely, a rehabilitation unit might have a low turnover rate because the patients in that unit have a longer LOS. The bed turnover rate is a measure of the frequency of bed use. It demonstrates the net effect of changes in occupancy rate and LOS. (See chapter 5 for a discussion of LOS.)

Following are two formulas for determining bed turnover rate. The direct formula is:

$$\frac{\textit{Number of discharges (including deaths) for a period}}{\textit{Average bed count during the period}}$$

The indirect formula is:

$$\frac{\textit{Occupancy Rate} \times \textit{Number of days in a period}}{\textit{Average length of stay}}$$

Although there is no universal agreement on the most accurate formula, administrators of short-stay hospitals are becoming increasingly interested in bed turnover rate as a measure of hospital services used, especially when related as a rate to occupancy and LOS. When occupancy goes up and LOS goes down, or vice versa, the bed turnover rate makes it easier to see the net effect of these changes.

Turnover rates can be used in comparing one facility with another or in comparing utilization rates for different time periods or for different units of the same facility. For example, the occupancy rate for one hospital can be essentially the same in two time periods, but the turnover rate may be lower because of a longer LOS in one time period. In other words, bed turnover rate can be a measure of intensity of utilization.

Exercise 4.7 displays both formulas and yields basically the same turnover rate for a short-stay hospital.

Exercise 4.7

**Community Hospital
Annual Statistics 20XX
Non-leap year
200 beds**

Patients discharged and died: 6,500
Average length of stay: 9 days
Bed occupancy rate: 80 percent

1. Apply the direct formula for the turnover rate. Round to one decimal place.

2. Apply the indirect formula for the turnover rate. Round to one decimal place.

Answers:

Turnover rate (direct formula):

Turnover rate (indirect formula):

Chapter 4 Test

A hospital compiled the following annual statistics for 20XX: (non-leap year)

**Community Hospital
Annual Statistics, 20XX**

	Inpatient Service Days	Bed Count
January–June	32,785	175
July–December	34,986	200
December 31 only	201	200
Newborn	12,372	40

Select the correct answer to each of the following questions, rounding to one decimal place.

1. The inpatient occupancy rate (without newborns) for 20XX was:

    a. 18.5%
    b. 37.4%
    c. 98.7%
    d. 99.0%

Chapter 4 Test (continued)

2. The newborn bassinet occupancy rate for 20XX was:

   a. 80.4%
   b. 84.7%
   c. 84.8%
   d. 85.2%

3. The bed occupancy rate for December 31 was:

   a. 77.1%
   b. 92.5%
   c. 100.0%
   d. 100.5%

The following table is a report of the first quarter of 20XX (January–March) from a 450-bed medical center regarding its insurance categories. Round all to one decimal place. This is a non-leap year. Use this table to answer #4, 5, and 6.

Community Medical Center
Inpatient Service Days and Number of Discharges
by Insurance Category
January–March, 20XX

Insurance Category	Inpatient Service Days	Number of Discharges
Third-party Contracts	4,859	666
Medicare	7,249	1,204
Medicaid	12,365	1,925
County Coverage	4,320	792
Private Pay	3,465	321
No Insurance	1,589	289
Total	**33,847**	**5,197**

4. Calculate the occupancy rate for:

   a. total
   b. Medicare
   c. private pay

5. Using the direct formula, calculate the bed turnover rate for:

   a. total
   b. Medicare
   c. private pay

6. What is the total average daily census for this period of time?

(continued on next page)

Chapter 4 Test (continued)

7. The following table is a report of the annual inpatient service days of Community Hospital for 20XX. The hospital has an inpatient bed count of 210 and a bassinet count of 30. Calculate (round to one decimal place) the percentage of occupancy for each month for adults/children and for newborns. This is a non-leap year.

Community Hospital
Annual Statistics, 20XX

| | Inpatient Service Days | | Percentage of Occupancy | |
Month	Adult/Children	Newborn	Adult/Children	Newborn
January	4,682	752		
February	4,798	798		
March	4,626	701		
April	1,876	688		
May	4,768	724		
June	4,591	743		
July	4,423	825		
August	4,234	796		
September	4,394	802		
October	4,412	865		
November	4,691	921		
December	4,832	912		
Total				

Chapter 5
Length of Stay

Objectives

At the conclusion of this chapter, you should be able to:

- Define the terms length of stay and discharge days
- Compute the length of stay for one patient based on data provided
- Calculate the total length of stay for a group of discharged patients
- Compute average length of stay
- Compute the average length of stay for newborns
- Describe a leave of absence day and identify when it is used in calculations

Length of Stay

Length of stay (LOS) is the number of calendar days a patient stays in the hospital, from admission to discharge. The healthcare facility uses LOS data in utilization management. **Utilization management** is a program that evaluates the facility's efficiency in providing necessary services in the most cost-effective manner, including LOS, while also evaluating the level of care required. Its goal is to eliminate over- and underutilization of services. Part of the utilization management process involves reviewing LOS for continued medical necessity. For example, is it more appropriate to continue to treat the patient in an acute care facility or to transfer the patient to a subacute or rehabilitation facility?

LOS data also are used in financial reporting, for example, to compare patients within the same Medicare Severity Diagnosis Related Group (MS-DRG). A particular MS-DRG **average length of stay** (ALOS) can be compared to the overall healthcare facility's MS-DRG ALOS to determine whether there are too many extreme values, or outliers. LOS data for patients with the same diagnosis or procedure treated by various physicians are compared to evaluate any extremes. For example, it is important for hospital administration to be aware of physician differences in LOS because these may be indicative of different types of treatment for the same condition by different physicians.

Discharge Days

Chapter 3 introduced the concept of inpatient service days, which are compiled while the patient is hospitalized. This chapter discusses **discharge days**, which are days compiled after the patient has been discharged from the hospital. Other terms for length of stay include **days of stay**, **inpatient days of stay**, and **duration of inpatient hospitalization**.

A discharge occurs at the end of the patient's hospital stay. Discharges include deaths, so the term *discharge* may refer to both patients who leave the hospital alive and those who have died. Often patients are transferred to other facilities to continue their care. Hospital staff may refer to these patients as transfers but they are counted as discharges.

In general, every day that a patient is in the hospital is counted as a day except the day of discharge. The LOS for one patient is determined by subtracting the **admission date** from the **discharge date** *when the patient is admitted and discharged within the same month*. The day of admission is counted in computing the number of discharge days or LOS, but the day of discharge is not.

For longer stays when the patient's stay extends beyond one or more months, days must be added to calculate the LOS.

> **Example:** For a patient admitted on January 30 and discharged on February 4, subtract January 30 from January 31 and add the 4 days in February ($31 - 30 = 1 + 4$ days in February = 5 days). The LOS is one day if the patient is admitted and discharged on the same day. These types of patients are also called admissions and discharges (A&Ds) or in and outs.

Table 5.1 shows how to calculate the LOS for a sampling of discharged patients.

Table 5.1.   Example LOS Calculation

Date Admitted	Date Discharged	Length of Stay
6/25	6/25	1 day
6/25	6/26	1 day (6/26 – 6/25 = 1 day)
6/25	6/30	5 days (6/30 – 6/25 = 5 days)
6/25	7/4	9 days (5 days in June + 4 days in July = 9 days)
6/25	8/4	40 days (5 days in June + 31 days in July + 4 days in August = 40 days)

Exercise 5.1

Calculate the LOS for the following discharged patients in an acute care facility.

Date Admitted	Date Discharged	Length of Stay
5/3	5/4	
7/2	7/12	
2/14	2/28	
3/25	4/15	
8/27	9/10	

Exercise 5.2

Calculate the LOS for the following discharged patients in this long-term care facility. Keep in mind that 2008 is a leap year.

Date Admitted	Date Discharged	Length of Stay
1/1/08	11/29/08	
4/17/07	12/01/08	
6/28/08	1/9/09	
2/1/08	4/8/09	
11/29/08	6/7/09	

It is possible to calculate LOS in an outpatient facility. For example, a patient arrived at 8:05 a.m. and was admitted to the examining room at 8:22 a.m. Because the hour is the same in both cases (8 a.m.), simply subtract the minutes (22 – 05 = 17 minutes). This patient waited 17 minutes before being admitted to the examining room. If a patient arrived at 8:05 a.m. and was taken into the examining room at 9:15, subtract the minutes first (15 – 5 = 10 minutes) and then subtract the hour (9 – 8 = 1). The patient waited 1 hour and 10 minutes.

If the number of minutes being subtracted is more than the original minutes, subtract 1 hour from the original number of hours and increase the number of original minutes by 60. Let's say a patient arrived at 1:11 p.m. and was taken to the examining room at 3:02 p.m. The original number of minutes (02) is less than the minutes being subtracted (11). So subtract 1 from the original number of hours (3 − 1 = 2) and add 60 to the number of minutes.

$$3:02 − 1:11 = 2:62 − 1:11 = 1:51.$$ The patient waited 1 hour and 51 minutes.

Handy Tip: This same technique can be used when calculating length of time spent in ambulatory care settings. For example, your administration may be interested in knowing the amount of time it takes to see patients in your facility.

Exercise 5.3

Calculate the time it takes to see patients in this physician's office.

Time Admitted	Time Seen by Physician	Time between Checking in at Reception and Being Seen by Physician
8:00 a.m.	8:17 a.m.	
1:22 p.m.	2:05 p.m.	
10:30 a.m.	11:43 a.m.	

Total Length of Stay

The **total length of stay** is the sum of the days' stay of any group of inpatients discharged during a specified period of time. Total length of stay also may be referred to as total discharge days. Although the total length of stay and inpatient service days may approximate each other over a long period of time, they are not interchangeable. The reason for this is that inpatient service days are counted concurrently and discharge days are counted after discharge.

Example: A patient hospitalized for a period beyond an entire year and into a second year (for example, a rehabilitation patient) would be credited with 365 inpatient service days at the end of the first year, but no discharge days. When the patient is discharged from the hospital in the second year, all the discharge days from admission to discharge are counted at that time, increasing the discharge days for the second year by at least 365.

If the patient stays in the hospital for two or more years (as happens in long-term facilities), all 730+ discharge days are assigned to one year in calculating the duration of inpatient hospitalization. These types of patients increase the number of discharge days for any year, making the total number much larger than inpatient service days for the same period.

Why calculate both inpatient days of service and total length of stay? Each is meaningful in its own right. Inpatient service days are useful in the analysis of current utilization of hospital facilities related to the entire hospital, a clinical unit, or a service department. They are used to compute various daily averages and occupancy ratios. The total length of stay can be used to analyze LOS for groups of discharged patients with similar characteristics such as age, disease, treatment, clinical service, or day of week admitted.

Exercise 5.4

Using the table below, calculate the LOS for each individual patient and then the total length of stay for the fifteen patients listed at Community Hospital.

All patients were discharged on 9/20/20XX.

**Community Hospital
Discharge List
September 20, 20XX**

Pt. Name	Age	Clinical Service	Admission Date	Length of Stay
Anderson	72	Medicine	9/18	
Bretz	43	Surgery	8/19	
Clemments	32	Obstetrics	9/18	
Dimmick	25	Obstetrics	9/18	
Erichson	98	Medicine	9/1	
Frye	67	Medicine	8/12	
Grell	43	Surgery	9/2	
Hallbauer	15	Obstetrics	9/19	
Imel	33	Medicine	9/17	
Jordan	51	Medicine	9/16	
Kirkpatrick	23	Obstetrics	9/17	
Locke	57	Surgery	8/3	
Miller	48	Surgery	8/31	
Nickel	59	Medicine	9/4	
Oller	63	Medicine	9/9	
Totals				

Finally, calculate the total length of stay for:

• Medicine service patients

• Surgery service patients

• Obstetrics service patients

(continued on next page)

Exercise 5.4 (continued)

- Patients 25 and younger
- Patients 26–40 years old
- Patients 41–55 years old
- Patients 56–70 years old or older
- Patients over age 70

Average Length of Stay

The average length of stay (ALOS) is the average number of days that inpatients discharged during the period under consideration stayed in the hospital. The formula for calculating ALOS is:

$$\frac{\textit{Total length of stay (discharge days)}}{\textit{Total discharges (including deaths)}}$$

In general, the inpatient LOS is decreasing. Several trends in healthcare have contributed to this reduction in ALOS, including managed care, home care, skilled nursing units in hospitals, and an increase in outpatient visits. Synonymous terms for ALOS include **average duration of hospitalization** and average stay.

The formula above does not include the ALOS for newborns. Most hospitals calculate the ALOS for newborns separately because newborns ordinarily stay the same length of time as their mothers. In addition, when compared to many other classifications of patients, normal newborn stays are relatively short. In contrast, newborn stays in the newborn intensive care unit tend to be quite long, sometimes months at a time. Therefore, inclusion of both mothers and newborns would distort the total ALOS.

Exercise 5.5

Complete the following exercises.

1. In February, Community Hospital reported 825 discharge days for adults and children and 96 discharge days for newborns. During the month, 158 adults and children and 32 newborns were discharged. Calculate (round to one decimal place) the ALOS for adults and children for the month of February.

2. Using the table in exercise 5.4, compute the ALOS for the group of patients between ages 41 and 55. The ALOS is 18.5 days. True or false?

   How would the median change the answer?

Exercise 5.5 (continued)

3. Using the report below from University Hospital for May 20XX, calculate (round to one decimal place) the ALOS for each service.

University Hospital
May, 20XX

Clinical Units	Discharges	Discharge Days	ALOS
Surgery	1,720	8,627	
Medicine	1,594	7,852	
Neurology	988	4,285	
Oncology	878	18,588	
Obstetrics/Gynecology	588	1,479	
Ophthalmology	385	1,154	
Orthopedics	651	9,321	
Pediatrics	358	2,841	
Psychiatry	156	4,697	
Rehabilitation	321	8,057	
Urology	89	183	
Total			

Average Newborn Length of Stay

As stated earlier, newborn LOS is usually calculated separately. The formula for calculating average newborn LOS is:

$$\frac{Total\ newborn\ discharge\ days}{Total\ newborn\ discharges\ (including\ deaths)}$$

Exercise 5.6

Using the table below, calculate (round to one decimal place) the ALOS for newborns in each month and then compute the annual ALOS.

University Hospital
Annual Newborn Discharge Statistics
20XX

Month	Newborn Discharges	Discharge Days	Newborn ALOS
January	95	238	
February	120	348	
March	112	347	
April	135	540	
May	142	454	
June	137	369	
July	176	616	
August	189	429	
September	207	601	
October	198	555	
November	152	501	
December	135	405	
Total			

Leave of Absence Days

Another data element that is significant in some hospitals is the number of leave of absence days. A **leave of absence** is a physician-authorized absence of an inpatient from a hospital or other facility for a specified period of time occurring after admission and prior to discharge. A **leave of absence day** is determined when the patient is not present at the census-taking hour. A leave of absence involves an overnight pass, or, more frequently given in longer-stay facilities, a weekend pass; thus, the patient would not be present when the census is taken.

Leave of absence data are important for administrative purposes as well as for the analysis of the services provided and care patterns. Leave of absence days are usually excluded or tabulated separately when computing bed occupancy, calculating inpatient service days, or preparing an inpatient census. Another issue with leave of absence days is that insurance companies generally do not pay for days outside the hospital. Thus, if the days are being used in conjunction with financial data, they may need to be separated from the actual days in the hospital. However, they are included when considering discharge days and computing ALOS. Hospitals that generally have longer lengths of stay, such as a rehabilitation, mental health, or chronic care hospital, will use the leave of absence day as a way for the patient to adjust to time away from the facility, so it is considered to be part of the patient's treatment. If the leave of absence is not considered part of the patient treatment, the physician may elect to discharge and then readmit the patient rather than grant a leave of absence.

Exercise 5.7

Using the statistics in the tables below, determine the following calculations for Community Hospital.

1. Compute the LOS for each of the patients in the table below.

    (Remember that 2008 was a leap year.)

Admitted	Discharged	LOS
1/12	1/31	
7/4	7/30	
1/1/2008	2/1/2009	
11/24	11/24	
6/19/2007	1/4/2009	

2. What is the total length of stay for this group of patients?

Using the statistics in the table below, determine the following calculations for Community Hospital. Round to one decimal place.

**Community Hospital
Annual Statistics, 20XX**

	Number of Discharges	Discharge Days
Total Adults and Children	15,987	92,725
Total Newborns	3,421	11,062
The following services are included in the above totals		
Medicine	11,644	51,201
Surgery	4,852	32,103
Obstetrics	2,912	10,483

Answers:

Adults and Children ALOS:

Newborns ALOS:

Medicine ALOS:

Surgery ALOS:

Obstetrics ALOS:

(continued on next page)

Exercise 5.7 (continued)

3. Compute the ALOS for adult and children patients.

4. Compute the ALOS for newborn patients.

5. Compute the ALOS for medicine patients.

6. Compute the ALOS for surgery patients.

7. Compute the ALOS for obstetrics patients.

8. Calculate the ALOS for the following Medicare patients.

Community Hospital
Medicare Discharge Statistics
July, 20XX

Unit	Medicare Discharges	Medicare Discharge Days	ALOS
Medicine	325	2,375	
Surgery	175	2,103	
Rehabilitation	298	4,179	
Skilled Nursing	305	6,588	

Chapter 5 Test

Last month, Community Hospital compiled the discharge statistics shown in the table on page 67. Notice that the last three days are missing. Prepare a spreadsheet on a software program and enter the information from the chart. Then use the discharge lists for May 29, 30, and 31 to enter the missing data into the appropriate columns for medicine, surgery, obstetrics, and newborn discharged patients and their corresponding discharge days.

Chapter 5 Test (continued)

Finally, compute the ALOS for medicine service, surgery service, OB service, and NB service and then compute the ALOS for adults and children (medicine, surgery, and OB).

**Community Hospital
Discharge List
May 29, 20XX**

Patient Name	Age	Service	Admission Date	LOS
Andres, Michael	74	Medicine	5-20	9
Barty, Stephen	43	Surgery	5-18	11
Christenson, Andrea	27	OB	5-27	2
Christenson, Baby Boy	NB	NB	5-27	2
Denison,William	51	Surgery	5-9	20
Henry, Christopher	76	Surgery	5-15	14
Jackson, Michelle	19	OB	5-26	3
Katon, Marie	39	OB	5-27	2
Williamson, Baby Boy	NB	NB	5-24	5

**Community Hospital
Discharge List
May 30, 20XX**

Patient Name	Age	Service	Admission Date	LOS
Adams, Paul	43	Medicine	5-26	4
Butler, Thomas	56	Medicine	5-28	2
Carson, Johnnie	76	Surgery	5-25	5
Daniels, George	54	Medicine	5-27	3
George, Michael	23	Surgery	5-26	4
Hanson, Joyce	19	OB	5-28	2
Hanson, Baby Girl	NB	NB	5-28	2
Jacquinta, Marlene	20	OB	5-26	4
Jacquinta, Baby Boy	NB	NB	5-26	4
Kettison, Jack	39	Medicine	5-25	5

(continued on next page)

Chapter 5 Test (continued)

Katosh, Joseph	67	Medicine	5-27	3
Kettison, Mary	67	Surgery	5-27	3
Laytham, Clint	60	Surgery	5-27	3
Matson, Dorianne	67	Medicine	5-28	2
Nettleson, Andy	34	Surgery	5-26	4
Otto, Pierce	78	Medicine	5-27	3
Ransom, Jackson	45	Medicine	5-25	5
Springer, Mary	56	Surgery	5-28	2
Tatum, Neal	34	Surgery	5-28	2
Wallace, Mattie	29	OB	5-30	1
Zininsky, Maureen	22	OB	5-29	1

**Community Hospital
Discharge List
May 31, 20XX**

Patient Name	Age	Service	Admission Date	LOS
Allan, Randy	42	Medicine	5-26	4
Banta, Janet	43	Medicine	5-25	6
Cox, David	78	Surgery	5-29	2
Dunning, Stephen	12	Surgery	5-28	3
Epp, Melvin	56	Medicine	5-24	7
Farmer, Jaimie	23	OB	5-28	3
Farmer, Baby Girl	NB	NB	5-28	3
Finney, G. W.	55	Surgery	5-27	4
Fry, Benedict	38	Surgery	5-28	3
Girard, Katherine	37	Medicine	5-29	2
Halford, Harold	55	Surgery	5-28	3
Kilpatrick, Susan	19	OB	5-28	3
Kilpatrick, Baby Boy	NB	NB	5-28	3
Martindale, Amanda	23	OB	5-28	3
Martindale, Baby Boy	NB	NB	5-28	3
McLoughlin, Baby Boy	NB	NB	5-27	4
Nachtigall, Brian	27	Medicine	5-27	4
Niazi, Baby Boy	NB	NB	5-27	4
Poepperling, Wanda	65	Medicine	5-28	3
Trotman, Baby Girl	NB	NB	5-30	1

Chapter 5 Test (continued)

Community Hospital
Student Name
May, 20XX

Date	Medicine No. Pts.	Medicine Disch Days	Surgery No. Pts.	Surgery Disch Days	Obstetrics No. Pts.	Obstetrics Disch Days	Subtotal No. Pts.	Subtotal Disch Days	Newborn No. Pts.	Newborn Disch Days	Total No. Pts.	Total Disch Days
1-May	12	36	5	23	2	8			3	12		
2-May	8	40	2	25	5	16			6	23		
3-May	6	36	8	80	3	10			3	10		
4-May	4	21	4	23	1	4			1	4		
5-May	11	47	3	42	4	10			4	10		
6-May	15	77	5	23	3	7			2	5		
7-May	6	52	7	56	2	5			3	7		
8-May	5	71	9	123	6	13			5	10		
9-May	8	63	1	4	3	9			2	13		
10-May	9	72	4	26	2	6			3	9		
11-May	7	34	9	112	3	8			3	8		
12-May	2	9	3	27	1	2			1	2		
13-May	5	28	4	16	2	5			1	3		
14-May	4	29	6	119	2	7			2	7		
15-May	9	26	8	95	2	6			2	6		
16-May	7	45	4	81	4	8			5	11		
17-May	6	37	2	15	3	8			3	8		
18-May	4	52	9	37	3	10			2	10		
19-May	8	63	3	37	2	6			3	9		
20-May	3	29	5	23	1	3			0	0		
21-May	5	35	8	78	4	9			4	9		
22-May	5	34	4	32	2	4			3	8		
23-May	8	53	1	5	3	6			3	6		
24-May	7	26	2	62	2	4			2	4		
25-May	2	23	3	42	4	12			2	7		
26-May	3	23	4	53	2	5			3	9		
27-May	5	25	2	10	3	10			4	11		
28-May	9	38	6	75	1	3			2	8		
29-May												
30-May												
31-May												
Totals	**183**	**1124**	**131**	**1344**	**75**	**204**	**0**	**0**	**77**	**229**		

Chapter 6
Death (Mortality) Rates

Objectives

At the conclusion of this chapter, you should be able to:

- Define and calculate the following death rates: gross, net, postoperative, anesthesia, maternal, newborn, and fetal

- Calculate the case fatality rate

- Differentiate between operation and procedure

- Define cancer mortality and calculate its rate

Death Rates

The **death rate** is the proportion of inpatient discharges that end in death, usually expressed as a percentage. The **hospital death rate** is defined as the number of inpatient deaths for a given period of time divided by the total number of live discharges and deaths for the same time period. A synonymous term for hospital death rate is **gross death rate**.

Death rates have always been important information for health agencies and hospitals in evaluating the quality of medical care. Death rate information is used by a variety of industries in addition to healthcare. For example, the automobile industry uses death rate information to determine the likelihood of drivers and/or passengers dying in some car models compared to others. Handgun advocates look at death rates to determine the likelihood of someone dying a violent death while using a firearm. Organizations such as the American Heart Association, the American Cancer Association, and other groups are interested in looking at death rates to help bring attention to their causes. Researchers use death rates to show causes of death in certain populations. All this information can help improve the quality of medical care given to patients.

An interesting article in the *Journal of the American Medical Association* calling for more emphasis on a new medical specialty—intensive care specialists, or intensivists—showed that having such intensive care experts could reduce death rates. The study showed that high numbers of intensivists was associated with lower hospital mortality and lower ICU mortality (Pronovost et al. 2002). The patients cared for by intensivists had reduced intensive care unit (ICU) and hospital death rates and lengths of stay (LOS). Health information management (HIM) practitioners—and anyone else who relies on statistical information—must remember that numbers count, not only in reports and records, but also in the human equation.

Death rate data also are important in helping public health agencies plan for health services. For example, the **Centers for Medicare and Medicaid Services** (CMS) publishes information on death rates among Medicare patients, specific ethnic groups, and patients in particular diagnosis categories, to name a few. Some years ago, CMS published a report for each hospital on Medicare deaths. Initially, the CMS **mortality** data received a great deal of media coverage and caused concern in facilities because of the high percentages reported. Moreover, the report created confusion about definitions and interpretation of the data. Hospitals were permitted to correct the data, and since the initial releases, the report format has been modified. This demonstrates the importance of the HIM practitioner's need to understand death rates. HIM practitioners must understand basic death rates and be ready to calculate or verify other data pertaining to mortality.

Gross (Hospital) Death Rate

In computing hospital death rates, the concept of number of occurrences versus number of times something could have occurred still applies. That is, every patient discharged from the hospital could possibly have died. Of course, this does not happen, but it is still a statistical possibility. Therefore, the formula for calculating the hospital death rate (gross death rate) is the number of patient deaths divided by the number of patient discharges (including deaths), as shown below:

$$\frac{Number\ of\ inpatient\ deaths\ (including\ NB)\ in\ a\ period\ \times 100}{Number\ of\ discharges\ (including\ A\&C\ and\ NB\ deaths)\ in\ the\ same\ period}$$

Example: If a hospital had five deaths and 400 discharges for a month, the gross death rate would be:

$$\frac{(5\times100)}{400}=1.25\%$$

This concept can be explored more specifically by means of the formula referred to as the **case fatality rate:**

$$\frac{Number\ of\ people\ who\ die\ of\ a\ disease\ in\ a\ specified\ period\ \times\ 100}{Number\ of\ people\ who\ have\ the\ disease}$$

Using the example of patients with severe acute respiratory syndrome (SARS), every patient discharged with the diagnosis of SARS has the potential to die. Thus, the formula is:

$$\frac{Number\ of\ patients\ with\ SARS\ who\ died\ \times\ 100}{Number\ of\ patients\ discharged\ with\ SARS\ diagnosis}$$

If a hospital had 20 influenza discharges last year and six deaths, the death rate would be:

$$\frac{(6\times100)}{20}=30.00\%$$

If 20 heart transplant patients were discharged and two died, the calculation would be:

$$\frac{(2\times100)}{20}=10.00\%$$

Example: The case fatality rate can be used to examine the death rates by physician. If Dr. Smith discharged 400 patients and 33 died, the formula would be:

$$\frac{(33\times100)}{400}=8.25\%$$

Guidelines for Calculating Death Rate

In calculating death rates, the following guidelines should be considered:

- Death is a type of discharge or **disposition**. Any data representing total discharges include deaths for that period. Thus, deaths are always assumed to be included in the total discharges in the denominator unless otherwise specified.

- If deaths of **newborn** inpatients are included in the numerator, all discharges of newborn inpatients must be included in the denominator. Ordinarily, newborns are included in the gross death rate unless a facility chooses to calculate their death rate separately.

- Patients who are **dead on arrival** (DOA) are not included in the gross death rate because DOAs are not admitted to the hospital.

- Patients who die in the emergency services department are not included in the gross death rate because they were not admitted to the hospital.

- Patients who die in the hospital while outpatients are not included in the gross death rate.

- **Fetal deaths** are not included in the hospital death rate but are calculated separately.

- Because death rates are ordinarily small, the calculation is usually carried out to three decimal places and rounded down to two places.

- It is a good idea to put a zero in front of the decimal (for example, 0.23%) to show the casual observer that the rate is less than one percent.

Exercise 6.1

Using the data below, calculate (round to two decimal places) the gross death rate at Community Hospital for May.

Community Hospital
May 20XX Data

Total adult and children discharges	540
Total adult and children deaths	9
Total newborn discharges	62
Total newborn deaths	1

Answer:

Exercise 6.2

The table below is a sample report for a hospital showing the discharges and deaths for the last quarter of the year. Notice that this report lists the patient discharges and deaths by physicians on the medical staff. Calculate the death rates for each physician and the total for this quarter (round to two decimal places). Deaths are not included in the discharges.

Community Hospital
October–December 20XX
Discharges and Deaths–Total Hospital Services

Physician Number	No. of Discharges	No. of Deaths	Gross Death Rate
Dr. 097	47	3	
Dr. 123	107	4	
Dr. 256	9	1	
Dr. 372	85	4	
Dr. 431	119	6	
Dr. 537	76	2	
Dr. 638	98	4	
Dr. 725	55	3	
Dr. 800	117	1	
Dr. 901	132	8	
Total			

Handy Tip: You may notice when computing your rates that sometimes your answer may be a whole number, such as 6% or there may be a zero in the hundredths place as in 6.1%. When asked to compute to two decimal places, always add the zeros. Your answer would read 6.00% and 6.10%.

Net Death Rate

Various reporting or accrediting agencies sometimes request the **net death rate**, also referred to as the **institutional death rate**. Historically, hospital inpatient deaths were classified as those that occurred less than 48 hours after admission and those deaths that occurred 48 hours or more after admission. The net death rate excludes deaths under 48 hours and is less than the gross death rate.

The net death rate came into use because it was felt that healthcare providers should not be held accountable for a death that occurred within less than 48 hours because they would not have had enough time to directly affect the patient's condition; only emergency treatment could be provided during this period of time. However, with the technology available today, many authorities believe this concept is no longer valid. The formula for calculating the net death rate is:

$$\frac{Total\ number\ of\ inpatient\ deaths\,(including\ NB)\ minus\ deaths < 48\ hours\ for\ a\ given\ period \times 100}{Total\ number\ of\ discharges\,(including\ NB\ deaths)\ minus\ deaths < 48\ hours\ from\ the\ same\ period}$$

Example: Last month, Community Hospital had 155 discharges, including eight deaths. Three of the deaths were patients who were in the hospital less than 48 hours. The net death rate would be calculated as follows:

$$\frac{(8-3)\times100}{(155-3)} = \frac{500}{152} = 3.29\%$$

Exercise 6.3

Using the data in the table below, calculate (round to two decimal places) the net death rate at Community Hospital for October. Discharges do not include deaths.

Community Hospital
October 20XX Data

Total adult and children discharges	307
Total adult and children deaths	5
Deaths < 48 hours	1
Deaths ≥ 48 hours	4
Total newborn discharges	62
Total newborn deaths	2
Deaths < 48 hours	1
Deaths ≥ 48 hours	1

Answer:

Exercise 6.4

Using the information in the table below, calculate (round to two decimal places) the net death rate for each service and the total net death rate at Community Hospital for September. In this exercise deaths are included in the discharges.

**Community Hospital
September 20XX Data**

Service	No. of Discharges	Deaths < 48 hours	Deaths ≥ 48 hours	Net Death Rate
Medicine	265	3	7	
Surgery	237	1	2	
Psychiatric	92	1	1	
Rehabilitation	42	1	3	
Total				

Postoperative Death Rate

The **postoperative death rate**, also called the **surgical death rate**, refers to the number of deaths occurring after an operation has been performed. Standard instructions for computing the postoperative death rate involve the ratio of deaths within 10 days after surgery to the total number of patients operated on during that period.

In appendix B of this book, a **surgical operation** is defined as one or more surgical procedures performed at one time for one patient via a common approach or for a common purpose. A **surgical procedure** is any single, separate, systematic process upon or within the body that can be complete in itself; is normally performed by a physician, dentist, or other licensed practitioner; can be performed either with or without instruments; and is performed to restore disunited or deficient parts, remove diseased or injured tissues, extract foreign matter, assist in obstetrical delivery, or aid in diagnosis.

The formula for calculating the postoperative death rate is:

$$\frac{Total\ number\ of\ deaths\ (within\ 10\ days\ after\ surgery) \times 100}{Total\ number\ of\ patients\ who\ were\ operated\ on\ for\ the\ period}$$

However, some healthcare practitioners question the usefulness of this calculation in evaluating the effectiveness of a hospital's medical care. Thus, rather than compute a total postoperative death rate, some hospitals evaluate the relationship of deaths following specific operations (for example, cholecystectomies or coronary artery bypass grafts).

Handy Tip: The standard formula for a rate applies here as well. All individuals who have surgery have the potential to die. The only difference here is that convention places a time limit of 10 days. After 10 days, concerns other than the surgery may cause the death of a patient. The denominator includes the patients operated on and not the number of operations because one patient may have several operations during a hospital stay.

Exercise 6.5

Using the information in the table below, calculate (round to two decimal places) the postoperative death rate for each surgeon at Community Hospital between January and March.

Community Hospital
January–March 20XX
Number of Surgery Patients and Deaths, by Surgeon

Physician Number	No. of Surgery Patients	No. of deaths within 10 days after surgery	Postoperative Death Rate
Dr. 102	180	4	
Dr. 237	120	2	
Dr. 391	60	1	
Dr. 518	65	1	
Dr. 637	98	5	
Dr. 802	32	3	
Dr. 900	64	1	

Exercise 6.6

Using the information in the table that follows, calculate (round to two decimal places) the postoperative death rate at Community Hospital during April.

Community Hospital
April 20XX Data
Surgery Service

Discharges	376
Deaths	6
Within 10 days of surgery	4
After 10 days of surgery	2
Number of operations	383
Number of patients operated on	370

Answer:

Exercise 6.7

Using the information in the table below, calculate (round to two decimal places) the postoperative death rate at Community Hospital for each Medicare Severity Diagnosis Related Group (MS-DRG) listed for July through December and the total for this semiannual period.

Community Hospital
July–December 20XX
Selected MS-DRGs—Postoperative Deaths
Number of Surgery Patients and Deaths
Surgery Service

MS-DRG	MS-DRG Title	No. of Surgery Patients	No. of deaths within 10 days after surgery	Postoperative Death Rate
338	Appendectomy w complicated principal diag w MCC	8	1	
327	Stomach, esophageal & duodenal proc w CC	67	2	
005	Liver transplant w MCC or intestinal transplant	17	6	
139	Salivary gland procedures	5	1	
405	Pancreas, liver & shunt procedures w MCC	54	3	
625	Thyroid, parathyroid & thyroglossal procedures w MCC	195	2	
736	Uterine & adnexa proc for ovarian or adnexal malignancy w MCC	132	5	
217	Cardiac valve & oth maj cardiothoracic proc w card cath w CC	201	3	
239	Amputation for circ sys disorders exc upper limb & toe w MCC	8	3	
469	Major joint replacement or reattachment of lower extremity w MCC	132	4	
Totals				

Anesthesia Death Rate

The traditional definition of **anesthesia death rate** is the ratio of deaths caused by anesthetic agents during a specified period to the number of anesthetics administered. Because anesthesia deaths occur infrequently, some hospitals might choose, instead, to evaluate the relationship between a death and a specific anesthetic for a special study.

There are three major types of anesthesia: general, regional, and local. General anesthesia puts the entire body to sleep. It is given intravenously or inhaled. Regional anesthesia removes the ability to feel any pain or sensations in a specific region of the body. This generally involves an injection of a local anesthetic agent around major nerves or the spinal cord. Spinal and epidural anesthesia and peripheral nerve blocks are a type of regional anesthesia and are used in many operations on specific portions of the body. Local anesthesia numbs a small area of the body. This involves an injection of an anesthetic.

The formula for calculating the anesthesia death rate is:

$$\frac{Total\ deaths\ caused\ by\ anesthetic\ agents \times 100}{Total\ number\ of\ anesthetics\ administered}$$

Example: If anesthetics were given 3,000 times to surgical patients and one patient death was attributed to anesthesia during the past year, the anesthesia death rate would be computed as follows:

$$\frac{(1 \times 100)}{3,000} = 0.03\%$$

Handy Tip: The fact that anesthesia deaths occur infrequently is reason to always check the placement of the decimal point in calculations of anesthesia death rates.

Exercise 6.8

Using the information in the table below, calculate (round to two decimal places) the anesthesia death rate for University Hospital for July through December.

University Hospital
July–December, 20XX
Surgery Service

Discharges	1,326
Deaths:	46
Within 10 days	14
After 10 days	32
Number of operations	1,329
Number of patients operated on	1,320
Number of anesthetics administered	1,326
Number of deaths due to anesthetic agents	4

Answer:

Exercise 6.9

Using the information in the table below, compute individually (round to two decimal places) the number of deaths due to the administration of general, regional, and local anesthesia.

University Hospital
July–December 20XX
Surgery Service

Discharges	1,326
Deaths	46
Within 10 days	14
After 10 days	32
Number of operations	1,329
Number of patients operated on	1,320
Number of anesthetics administered	1,326
General anesthesia	663
Regional anesthesia	530
Local anesthesia	133
Number of deaths due to anesthetic agents	4
General anesthesia	2
Regional anesthesia	1
Local anesthesia	1

Answer:

Maternal Death Rate

A **maternal death** is defined as the death of any woman from any cause related to or aggravated by pregnancy or its management (regardless of duration or site of pregnancy, but not from accidental or incidental causes). An example of an accidental death would be a motor vehicle accident or a fall down a flight of stairs. An example of an incidental death would be a suicide or homicide.

Many healthcare facilities also differentiate between direct obstetric deaths and indirect obstetric deaths. A *direct obstetric death* is a death directly related to the pregnancy, for example, a patient who died after a C-section because of a nick to the uterine artery that resulted in hemorrhage. An *indirect obstetric death* is not directly due to obstetric causes, even though the physiologic effects of the pregnancy are partially responsible for the death. An example of an indirect obstetric death is diabetes. A pregnant woman can have **complications** of the diabetes that are aggravated by the pregnancy, but the cause of death is the diabetes and not the pregnancy.

Computing Maternal Death Rate

When computing the **maternal death rate**, hospitals usually classify only direct obstetric deaths as maternal deaths and include only those deaths that occur during hospitalization. Nonmaternal deaths (deaths resulting from accidental or incidental causes not related to pregnancy or its management) are not included. A woman who dies after an abortion is considered a maternal death, as is an obstetric patient who dies in the **prepartum** period (that is, the time period occurring before childbirth—some facilities refer to these as *antepartum* deaths) of a cause due to pregnancy. If the service classification system includes a breakdown of obstetrical discharges into delivered, aborted, not delivered, and **postpartum** (the time after childbirth), all these should be included in the total obstetrical discharges in the denominator of the formula (and in the numerator if the mother dies).

The formula for calculating the maternal death rate is:

$$\frac{\textit{Number of direct maternal deaths for a period} \times 100}{\textit{Number of obstetrical discharges (including deaths) for the period}}$$

Example: At one hospital, a mother died immediately after delivery. The hospital's annual obstetric/gynecology discharges are classified as: delivered, 5,000; aborted, 100; not delivered (prepartum), 200; and postpartum, 20.

Please note in this example that some patients are divided into prepartum (not delivered) and postpartum cases. A patient who comes into the hospital in labor but does not deliver and is discharged home is considered a prepartum patient; a patient who comes into the hospital after delivery with an infection of the C-section incision site is considered a postpartum patient.

The calculation of the hospital maternal mortality rate is:

$$\frac{(1 \times 100)}{(5,000 + 100 + 200 + 20)} = \frac{100}{5,320} = 0.018 = 0.02\%$$

Handy Tip: Just as with other death rates, the maternal death rate calculation is usually carried to three decimal places and then rounded to two places.

Computing Vital Statistics for Maternal Mortality Rate

As previously noted in chapter 1, researchers frequently use vital statistics information for public health and policy studies. Researchers use a number other than 100 in the numerator because they are not interested in determining percentages but, rather, the number of times something occurs in the population. For example, researchers may use 100,000 to determine how often something occurred per 100,000 people, 10,000 to determine how often it occurred per 10,000 people, and so on.

The following vital statistics formula for maternal mortality rate may be used in the United States:

$$\frac{\textit{Number of deaths attributed to maternal conditions during a period} \times 100,000}{\textit{Number of births during the period}}$$

Example: During the year, a women's hospital reported 1,205 **hospital live births** and two deaths after abortions. The vital statistics maternal mortality rate would be calculated as follows:

$$\frac{(2 \times 100,000)}{1,205} = \frac{200,000}{1,205} = 165.975 = 166 \text{ per } 100,000 \text{ births}$$

$$\frac{(2 \times 10,000)}{1,205} = \frac{20,000}{1,205} = 16.5975 = 16.6 \text{ per } 10,000 \text{ births}$$

$$\frac{(2 \times 1,000)}{1,205} = \frac{2,000}{1,205} = 1.65 = 1.7 \text{ per } 1,000 \text{ births}$$

Exercise 6.10

Using the information in the table below, calculate (round to two decimal places) Community Hospital's maternal death rate for April. These are all direct maternal deaths.

Community Hospital
April 20XX
Obstetrical Unit

Discharges	
Delivered	220
Aborted	2
Undelivered, prepartum	22
Undelivered, postpartum	15
Deaths	
Delivered	1
Aborted	1
Undelivered, prepartum	1
Undelivered, postpartum	2

Answer:

Exercise 6.11

Last month, The Women's Hospital reported 134 obstetrical discharges and four deaths. (The deaths are included in the discharges.) The causes of the four deaths were:

- Injuries due to abuse by husband
- Heroine overdose
- Hemorrhage after C-section due to severed uterine artery
- Pregnancy-induced hypertension

Calculate the direct maternal death rate (round to two decimal places) for this hospital.

Exercise 6.12

Using the annual statistics in the table below, calculate (round to two decimal places) the maternal death rate and the abortion death rate for University Hospital. These are all direct maternal deaths.

University Hospital
Annual Statistics 20XX
Obstetrical Service

Discharges:	
Delivered	903
Aborted	36
Undelivered, prepartum	85
Undelivered, postpartum	76
Deaths:	
Delivered	2
Aborted	1
Undelivered, prepartum	1
Undelivered, postpartum	1

Answer:

Exercise 6.12 (continued)

Deaths:

Delivered

Aborted

Undelivered, prepartum

Undelivered, postpartm

Newborn Mortality Rate

Statistical tabulations for vital events related to pregnancy and newborns can provide valuable information on reproductive health. They also can provide data on national and international trends.

The following definitions apply to infant deaths:

- **Neonatal death** refers to the death of a liveborn infant within the **neonatal period** of 27 days, 23 hours, and 59 minutes from the moment of birth.

- **Postneonatal death** refers to the death of a liveborn infant from 28 days of birth to the end of the first year of life (through 364 days, 23 hours, 59 minutes from the moment of birth).

- **Infant death** refers to the death of a liveborn infant at any time from the moment of birth to the end of the first year of life (through 364 days, 23 hours, 59 minutes from the moment of birth).

- **Perinatal death** is an all-inclusive term referring to both stillborn infants and neonatal deaths.

The formula for calculating the **newborn mortality rate** is:

$$\frac{\text{Total number of newborn deaths for a period} \times 100}{\text{Total number of newborn discharges (including deaths) for the period}}$$

Handy Tip: When computing newborn mortality rates, the answer should be carried out to at least three decimal places and rounded to two places. This is important because newborn death rates are also usually very small. When healthcare facilities report discharges, they typically include deaths in the discharge figures because a death is a type of a discharge.

Example: If a hospital had 2,000 newborn discharges and one newborn death in one year, its newborn mortality rate would be calculated as:

$$\frac{(1 \times 100)}{2,000} = 0.05\%$$

Computing Vital Statistics for Neonatal and Infant Mortality Rate

Researchers frequently use birth certificate data for public health and policy studies. Similar vital statistics formulas are used in the United States. Following are two examples of vital statistics formulas:

Neonatal mortality rate formula:

$$\frac{Number\ of\ neonatal\ deaths\ during\ a\ period \times 1{,}000}{Number\ of\ live\ births\ during\ the\ period}$$

Infant mortality rate formula:

$$\frac{Number\ of\ infant\ deaths\ (neonatal\ and\ postneonatal)\ during\ a\ period \times 1{,}000}{Number\ of\ live\ births\ during\ the\ period}$$

Example: If a hospital had 3,856 births, 3 newborn deaths, and 3,850 newborn discharges, the vital statistics neonatal mortality rate would be calculated as follows:

$$\frac{(3 \times 100)}{3{,}856} = \frac{3{,}000}{3{,}856} = 0.7780 = 0.8\ per\ 1{,}000$$

Exercise 6.13

Using the information in the table below, calculate (round to two decimal places) Community Hospital's annual newborn mortality rate. In this exercise, the deaths are included in the discharges.

Community Hospital
Annual Statistics 20XX
Newborn Service

Births	379
Newborn Deaths	1
Newborn Discharges	380

Answer:

Exercise 6.14

Using the information in the table below, calculate (round to two decimal places) the newborn death rate for February at Community Hospital. In this exercise, the deaths are included in the discharges.

Community Hospital
Newborn Unit
February 20XX

Births	32
Discharges	32
Deaths	1
Answer:	

Fetal Death Rate

A hospital fetal death is defined as a death prior to the complete expulsion or extraction from the mother (in a hospital facility) of a product of human conception (fetus and placenta) regardless of the duration of pregnancy. The death is indicated by the fact that after such expulsion or extraction, the fetus does not breathe or show any other evidence of life (for example, beating of the heart, pulsation of the umbilical cord, or definite movement of voluntary muscles). Typically, hospitals are required to report fetal deaths to a state agency. However, the reporting method varies according to individual state laws, statutes, and regulations.

Because fetal deaths are not considered patient deaths, they are not included in any other calculation of deaths but, instead, are calculated separately. Determination of whether to include fetal death data in a specific hospital's statistics requires an investigation of the facility's needs by hospital administration, medical staff, and reporting agencies. As with the other death rates, fetal deaths may be classified as:

- **Early fetal death**: Fewer than 20 weeks of gestation and a weight of 500 grams or less

- **Intermediate fetal death**: Twenty completed weeks of gestation (but less than 28 weeks) and a weight of 501 to 1,000 grams

- **Late fetal death**: Twenty-eight completed weeks of gestation and a weight of 1,001 grams or more

Both intermediate and late fetal deaths constitute what is commonly termed a **still-birth**. The formula for calculating the **fetal death rate** is:

$$\frac{\textit{Total number of intermediate and/or late fetal deaths for a period} \times 100}{\textit{Total number of live births} + \textit{Intermediate and late fetal deaths for the period}}$$

Example: During June, a hospital had 100 live births, one intermediate fetal death, and three late fetal deaths. To determine the fetal death rate for the hospital, the total number of intermediate and late fetal deaths (4) is multiplied by 100 and divided by the total number of live births and the intermediate and late fetal deaths (100 + 4). The calculation is as follows:

$$\frac{(4 \times 100)}{(100 + 4)} = \frac{400}{104} = 3.846\% = 3.85\%$$

Handy Tip: Keep in mind that the denominator in the fetal death rate formula does not include discharges. If you remember the formula for rates discussed in Chapter 2, that is, the number of times something actually happened in relation to the number of times it could have happened, it becomes clear that every birth could be a fetal death. And, be sure to include the intermediate and late fetal deaths in the denominator. Also remember that newborn births are the same as newborn admissions.

Exercise 6.15

Community Hospital reported the following statistics for the month of July. Calculate (round to two decimal places) the fetal death rate.

Community Hospital
July 20XX
Newborn Service

Live Births	29
Newborn discharges	32
Fetal Deaths:	
Early	1
Intermediate	2
Late	4
Answer:	

Exercise 6.16

Using the information in the table below, calculate (round to two decimal places) the newborn mortality rate and fetal death rate at Community Hospital for the year. In this exercise, deaths are included in the discharges.

Community Hospital
January–December 20XX
Newborn Service

Live Births	245
Newborn discharges	248
Newborn deaths	3
Fetal Deaths:	
Early	5
Intermediate	3
Late	1

Answers:
Newborn death rate:

Fetal death rate:

Cancer Mortality Rate

A **mortality rate** measures the risk of death for the cause under study in a defined population during a given time period. The National Center for Health Statistics collects data on all cancer deaths occurring in the United States and classifies them by sex, age, race, and cancer site so that mortality for a given time period can be determined for the entire country or selected areas.

The formula for calculating the **cancer mortality rate** for a population is:

$$\frac{Number\ of\ cancer\ deaths\ during\ a\ period \times 100}{Total\ number\ in\ population\ at\ risk}$$

Example: In 2005, 559,312 people died from cancer in the United States. The estimated 2005 census for the U.S. population was 296,410,404. The formula for calculating the cancer mortality rate per 100,000 people in 2005 would be:

$$\frac{Number\ of\ cancer\ deaths\ in\ 2005}{Population\ at\ risk}$$

Using the statistics provided here, the calculation would be as follows:

$$\frac{(559{,}312 \times 100{,}000)}{296{,}410{,}404} = 188.7 \text{ deaths per 100,000 population}$$

This is a **crude death rate** because it encompasses deaths from all forms of cancer for persons of all ages and races and of both sexes. In other words, it is based on the entire U.S. population. Specific rates can be calculated to describe risks for specific cancers in entire populations or specific subgroups of a population, such as age-specific rates or sex-specific rates.

Knowledge of healthcare statistics is an essential tool for cancer registrars. A cancer registrar is an individual who is responsible for maintaining records and reporting information about cancer patients. Cancer registries were developed as organized programs in hospitals to collect information about cancer patients. Hospital and other cancer registry data are reported to population-based (central or regional) registries.

When you are calculating the cancer death rate in your own facility, use the formula for a rate—that is the number of deaths from a specific diagnosis of cancer divided by the number of discharges of that same diagnosis of cancer.

Exercise 6.17

Using the information given in the table below from Community Hospital's Cancer Registry, calculate (round to two decimal places) the death rates for each type of cancer and the total for this annual period. Deaths are included in the discharges.

Community Hospital
Cancer Registry Annual Report
Selected Cancers Reported
20XX

Type of Cancer	No. of Discharges	No. of Deaths	Death Rate
Prostate	23	6	
Breast	56	4	
Lung and Bronchus	28	9	
Colon/Rectum	39	2	
Uterus	36	5	
Urinary Bladder	15	2	
Non-Hodgkin's Lymphoma	21	6	
Melanoma of the Skin	23	5	
Kidney and Renal Pelvis	15	3	
Ovary	12	5	
Total			

Exercise 6.18

Using the statistics in the table below from a multihospital system, calculate (round to two decimal places) the death rate for each hospital listed and for the entire healthcare system. In this exercise, the deaths are included in the discharges.

**Community Healthcare System
Annual Statistics 20XX**

Hospital	Discharges	Deaths	Death Rate
Urban Hospital	14,962	172	
Rural Hospital	5,403	107	
Psychiatric Hospital	1,243	6	
Rehabilitation Hospital	1,159	24	
Totals			

Chapter 6 Test

Using the data reported below for the past year, perform the calculations requested below. (Round these to two decimal places.)

Discharges (includes deaths)

Total adults and children	12,954
Total newborns	1,865

The following are included in the discharges:

OB delivered	1,871
OB aborted	125
OB undelivered, prepartum	20
OB undelivered, postpartum	32

Admissions

Total adults and children	13,023
Total live births	1,864

Deaths

Total adults and children	47
Total newborns	2

The following are included in the deaths:

Within 10 days postop	2
< 48 hours after admission	12
≥ 48 hours after admission	35
Anesthetic death	1

Obstetric deaths:

Undelivered, prepartum	1
Aborted	1

Fetal deaths:

Early	7
Intermediate	5
Late	2

Total patients operated on	4,533
Total anesthetics administered	4,533

(continued on next page)

Chapter 6 Test (continued)

1. The gross death rate is:
   a. 0.033%
   b. 0.33%
   c. 3.31%
   d. 33.10

2. The net death rate is:
   a. 0.25%
   b. 2.51%
   c. 0.025%
   d. 25.10%

3. The postoperative death rate is 0.05 percent. True or false?

4. What is the anesthesia death rate?

5. What is the maternal death rate?

6. What is the newborn mortality rate?

7. What is the fetal death rate?

8. The gross death rate excludes deaths that occur within 48 hours of admission. True or false?

9. According to standard instructions, deaths within 15 days after surgery are used to compute the postoperative death rate. True or false?

10. Anesthesia deaths occur frequently. True or false?

11. Which of the following deaths is also called the institutional death rate?
    a. Gross death rate
    b. Net death rate
    c. Postoperative death rate

12. What is the gestational age and gram weight for early fetal death, intermediate fetal death, and late fetal death?

Chapter 6 Test (continued)

Use the information in the table below to answer questions 13 through 19. In these exercises, the deaths are included in the discharges and deaths occurring in less than 48 hours and postop deaths are included in the deaths.

Community Hospital
Annual Statistics 20XX

Service	Discharges	Deaths	< 48 hours	Postop
Medicine	1,375	84	13	0
Surgery	1,098	22	9	3
Obstetrics	632	1	0	0
Newborn	633	1	1	0
Psychiatric	321	1	0	0
Rehabilitation	291	16	0	0
Totals				

Additional information

Anesthetics administered	1,094
Anesthetic deaths	1
Patients operated on	1,094
Total livebirths	633
Fetal deaths:	
Early	7
Intermediate	4
Late	1

13. What is the gross death rate?

14. What is the net death rate?

15. What is the postoperative death rate?

16. What is the anesthesia death rate?

17. What is the maternal death rate?

18. What is the newborn mortality rate?

19. What is the fetal death rate?

(continued on next page)

Chapter 6 Test (continued)

Using the information in the table below, calculate the death rates for University Hospital's Cancer Registry for each of the cancers reported and the total for this annual period. In these exercise, the deaths are included in the discharges.

University Hospital
Cancer Registry Annual Report
Selected Cancers Reported
20XX

Type of Cancer	No. of Discharges	No. of Deaths	Death Rate
Prostate	236	16	
Breast	368	24	
Lung and Bronchus	281	29	
Colon/Rectum	397	12	
Uterus	130	5	
Urinary Bladder	101	2	
Non-Hodgkin's Lymphoma	203	16	
Melanoma of the skin	239	5	
Kidney and Renal Pelvis	105	13	
Ovary	98	15	
Total			

Chapter 7
Hospital Autopsies and Autopsy Rates

Objectives

At the conclusion of this chapter, you should be able to:

- Define the terms autopsy, hospital inpatient autopsy, hospital autopsy, and autopsy rate

- Define and differentiate between a coroner and medical examiner

- Define a coroner's case and determine when it would be included in a hospital's autopsy rate

- Compute the following autopsy rates: gross, net, adjusted hospital, newborn, and fetal

Autopsy

An **autopsy** is the examination of a dead body to determine the cause of death. Autopsies are performed in order to educate physicians and allied health professionals. An autopsy can be performed on the entire body or a particular body organ. Another name for autopsy is **necropsy** or **postmortem** (after death) **examination.** Autopsies are generally performed by either a hospital pathologist or a physician on the medical staff who has been delegated this responsibility. They are usually performed in the hospital **morgue**, but in the case of small hospitals that do not have a morgue, the body may be removed to an off-site lab or a funeral home for the autopsy.

Gross Autopsy Rate

The **autopsy rate** is the proportion of deaths that are followed by the performance of an autopsy. A **gross autopsy rate** is the ratio during any given period of time of all inpatient autopsies to all inpatient deaths. The rate is customarily reported as a percentage. Again, the concept of a rate applies here: the number of times something actually happened compared to the number of times it could have happened. Statistically speaking, every patient who dies could be autopsied. Typically, newborn autopsies are included in the gross autopsy rate but may be calculated separately as determined by the hospital's administration or medical staff committee.

The formula for calculating the gross autopsy rate is:

$$\frac{Total\ autopsies\ on\ inpatient\ deaths\ for\ a\ period \times 100}{Total\ inpatient\ deaths\ for\ the\ period}$$

Example: During July, Community Hospital discharged 918 patients. The hospital had 32 deaths (including newborns) and performed 9 autopsies. Using the formula given above, the gross autopsy rate is determined to be 28.13 percent, as follows:

$$\frac{(9 \times 100)}{32} = \frac{900}{32} = 28.13$$

Handy Tip: Although death rates are usually small, autopsy rates can be fairly large.

Exercise 7.1

In a one-month period, a 360-bed hospital with 20 bassinets reported 24 inpatient deaths. The medical staff performed 6 autopsies. The gross autopsy rate is 32.50 percent. True or false?

Exercise 7.2

Using the information in the table below, calculate (round to two decimal places) the gross death rate, the net death rate, and the gross autopsy rate for Community Hospital for the time period.

**Community Hospital
Hospital Statistics
January–June 20XX**

Total inpatient discharges (including deaths)	378
Total inpatient deaths	18
(< 48 hours)	(3)
Total autopsies	5

Answers:

Gross death rate:

Net death rate:

Gross autopsy rate:

Net Autopsy Rate

The **net autopsy rate** is the ratio during any given period of time of all inpatient autopsies to all inpatient deaths, minus any unautopsied coroners' or medical examiners' cases. The formula for net autopsy rate differs slightly from the formula for gross autopsy rate in that it excludes bodies that have been removed by the coroner or medical examiner.

Certain types of deaths are reportable to the coroner of a particular jurisdiction. A **coroner** is the official (elected or appointed, physician or nonphysician) who is responsible for determining the cause, time, and manner of death in unattended, violent, or unexplained deaths. Coroners may also have other duties depending on their state. The word comes from the Old English word *corono,* which means "crown." The English crown originally appointed coroners.

In some areas of the country, the coroner has been replaced with a **medical examiner** (ME). The medical examiner is usually an appointed official who is a physician, commonly holding a specialty in pathology or forensic medicine. A body released to a coroner or medical examiner is not available for autopsy by the hospital pathologist.

The formula for calculating the net autopsy rate is:

$$\frac{\textit{Total autopsies on inpatient deaths for a period} \times 100}{\textit{Total inpatient deaths} - \textit{Unautopsied coroners' or medical examiners' cases}}$$

Example: During August, a hospital had 42 patient deaths and performed 14 autopsies. Two bodies were released to the county coroner for autopsy. Therefore, two cases are subtracted from the denominator because they were not autopsied by the hospital. Dividing the number of inpatient autopsies performed (14) by the total number of bodies available for autopsy (42 – 2 = 40) produces a net autopsy rate of 35 percent, as shown in the equation below.

$$\frac{(14 \times 100)}{(42-2)} = \frac{1,400}{40} = 35.0\%$$

Handy Tip: If the coroner or medical examiner requests the hospital pathologist perform the autopsy, it is included in the rate and not subtracted out because the case would not be unavailable for autopsy.

Exercise 7.3

Over the past year, University Hospital had 16,523 discharges, 288 inpatient deaths, and 185 autopsies. The bodies of 20 patients were released to the medical examiner for autopsy. Calculate (round to two decimal places) the gross death, gross autopsy, and net autopsy rates for University Hospital.

Answers:

Gross death rate:

Gross autopsy rate:

Net autopsy rate:

Handy Tip: The net autopsy rate will be higher than the gross autopsy rate because the denominator includes unautopsied coroners' or medical examiners' cases. Because there is a lower number of autopsies in the denominator, the rate will be higher.

Exercise 7.4

Using the information in the table below, calculate (round to two decimal places) the gross death, gross autopsy, and net autopsy rates for University Hospital. In this exercise, the deaths are included in the discharges.

**University Hospital
Quarterly Statistics
October–December 20XX**

Discharges:	
Adults and children	3,304
Newborn	826
Deaths:	
Adults and children	70
Newborn	2
Inpatient Autopsies	46
Coroner's cases (unavailable for autopsy)	5

Answers:

Gross death rate:

Gross autopsy rate:

Net autopsy rate:

Hospital Autopsies

A **hospital inpatient autopsy** is the postmortem examination that is ordinarily performed in a hospital facility on the body of an inpatient who died during hospitalization. In contrast, a **hospital autopsy** is the postmortem examination of the body of a person who has *at some time* been a hospital patient. Former inpatients may include emergency patients, outpatients, and home care patients.

When determining what autopsies to include in the **hospital autopsy rate**, the following guidelines apply:

- Hospital autopsies are usually performed by the facility pathologist. However, small hospitals do not always have a pathologist on staff, so responsibility for performing autopsies may be delegated to another physician.

- Normally, hospital autopsies are performed in hospitals. However, a small hospital or a specialized hospital (for example, obstetrical or psychiatric) may not have many deaths and thus may not be equipped with the necessary facilities to perform autopsies. In such cases, the autopsies are performed in another designated place.

- As a general rule, hospital autopsies are performed on deceased inpatients. However, because of the educational value of autopsies, former inpatients who were not in the hospital at the time of death may be considered for hospital autopsies. These individuals may include Emergency Services Department (ESD) patients, outpatients, and home care or hospice deaths. This is the only case where outpatients are included with inpatient statistics.

- Fetal autopsies are not included in the hospital autopsy rate because a fetus is not considered a patient.

- The essential components for a hospital autopsy are the following:

  — The autopsy must be performed by a staff pathologist or a delegated physician.

  — There must be a consent from the patient's next of kin or legal representative to perform an autopsy, which is filed in the medical record. The consent may be for a full body autopsy or a partial autopsy.

  — The autopsy report must be filed in the patient's health record.

  — The tissue specimens must be filed in the hospital laboratory along with the autopsy report.

Examples of hospital autopsy cases include:

- A patient dies in the hospital and is autopsied by the hospital's pathologist in the local morgue.

- A patient dies in the hospital, and one of the hospital's physicians is delegated to perform the autopsy in the absence of the staff pathologist.

- A former patient is pronounced dead on arrival (DOA) in the hospital's ESD, and the staff pathologist performs the autopsy.

Adjusted Hospital Autopsy Rate

The **adjusted hospital autopsy rate** is the proportion of hospital autopsies performed following the deaths of patients whose bodies are available for autopsy. Although many hospitals calculate the net autopsy rate for various surveys and external reports, the adjusted hospital autopsy rate is a more accurate indication of the hospital's resources for physician education because it includes all autopsies.

The formula for calculating the adjusted hospital autopsy rate is:

$$\frac{Total\ hospital\ autopsies \times 100}{Total\ number\ of\ deaths\ of\ hospital\ patients\ whose\ bodies\ are\ available\ for\ autopsy}$$

Patients whose bodies are **available for hospital autopsy** include:

- Inpatients (unless the bodies are removed from the hospital by legal authorities such as the coroner or medical examiner). However, if the hospital pathologist or delegated physician performs an autopsy while acting as an agent of the coroner or medical examiner, the autopsy is included in the numerator and the death in the denominator of the adjusted hospital autopsy rate formula.

- Other patients, including hospital home care patients, outpatients, and previous hospital patients who have died elsewhere and whose bodies have been made available for the performance of hospital autopsies.

Example: Community Hospital had 255 discharges in July, eight of which were deaths. The hospital pathologist performed three of the autopsies. During this period, two home care patients died and were brought to the hospital for autopsy. To determine the adjusted hospital autopsy rate, add all the hospital autopsies performed to determine the numerator (3 inpatients + 2 home care patients). The denominator contains all the inpatients and home care patients who died in July (8 + 2).

$$\frac{(3+2) \times 100}{(8+2)} = 50.0\%$$

Handy Tip: In the previous formulas, outpatients, ESD patients, and home care patients were not included with the inpatients. When calculating the adjusted hospital autopsy rate, the outpatients, ESD patients, and home care patients would be included if their bodies were autopsied by the hospital pathologist.

Exercise 7.5

Using the data in the table below, calculate (round to two decimal places) the gross death, gross autopsy, net autopsy, and adjusted hospital autopsy rates for University Hospital. In this exercise, the deaths are included in the discharges.

University Hospital
Annual Statistics
20XX

Discharges:	
Adults and children	12,924
Newborn	4,332
Deaths:	
Adults and children	345
Newborn	3
Deaths in the ESD and OPD*	15
Autopsies:	
Inpatient	159
ESD/OPD	14
Coroner's cases (unavailable for autopsy)	6

Answers:

Gross death rate:

Gross autopsy rate:

Net autopsy rate:

Adjusted hospital autopsy rate:

---

* ESD = Emergency Services Department; OPD = Outpatient Department

Exercise 7.6

Using the information in the table below, calculate (round to two decimal places) the adjusted hospital autopsy rate.

**Community Hospital
July Statistics**

Inpatient deaths	8
ESD deaths	3
Home health death	1
Inpatient autopsies	2
ESD autopsy	1
Home health autopsy	1
Coroner's cases (unavailable for autopsy)	1

Answer:

Adjusted hospital autopsy rate:

Exercise 7.7

In January, University Hospital had 23 inpatient deaths, 8 of which were autopsied. Of the 23 deaths, two were coroner's cases—one of which was autopsied by the hospital pathologist (included in the 8 autopsies), and one was removed to be autopsied by the coroner. In addition, the following cases were brought to the hospital to be autopsied: a former inpatient who died in a skilled nursing facility a month after discharge from the hospital; a child known to have congenital heart disease who died in the ESD; one patient who died in the outpatient department while he was getting lab work performed, and a former inpatient who died at home while under the hospital's home care department. Calculate (round to two decimal places) the adjusted hospital autopsy rate for University Hospital for this month.

Newborn Autopsy Rate

The **newborn autopsy rate** is the proportion of hospital autopsies performed following the deaths of newborns.

The formula for calculating the newborn autopsy rate is:

$$\frac{Newborn\ autopsies\ for\ a\ period \times 100}{Total\ newborn\ deaths\ for\ the\ period}$$

Example: Community Hospital had 27 births during the month of September. One newborn died shortly after birth and was autopsied. Applying the formula above, the correct newborn autopsy rate is 100 percent.

$$\frac{(1 \times 100)}{1} = 100.0\%$$

Exercise 7.8

Using the information in the table below, calculate (round to two decimal places) the newborn death rate and the newborn autopsy rate for University Hospital. In this exercise, the deaths are included in the discharges.

**University Hospital
Newborn Statistics**

Births	402
Discharges	398
Deaths	3
Autopsies	2

Answer:

Newborn death rate:

Newborn autopsy rate:

Exercise 7.9

In September 20XX, the newborn unit at Community Hospital reported four stillbirths and two newborn deaths. An autopsy was performed on one of the newborns and two stillbirths. Calculate (round to two decimal places) the newborn autopsy rate for September.

Answer:

Newborn autopsy rate:

Exercise 7.10

University Hospital reported the following quarterly statistics for January–March 20XX: 483 discharges, four newborn deaths, three stillbirths. There were two newborn autopsies. One newborn was born in a taxi on the way to the hospital, was admitted and later died. It was autopsied. One newborn was born at home and brought to the hospital and admitted. It also died and was autopsied. Calculate (round to two decimal places) University Hospital's newborn death rate and newborn autopsy rate. In this exercise, the deaths are included in the discharges.

Answer:

Newborn death rate:

Newborn autopsy rate:

Handy Tip: Remember that a newborn is an inpatient who was born in a hospital at the beginning of the current inpatient hospitalizations. A newborn born outside the hospital and then admitted is considered a pediatric admission.

Fetal Autopsy Rate

The **fetal autopsy rate** is the proportion of hospital autopsies performed following the deaths of intermediate and late fetal deaths.

The formula for the fetal autopsy rate is:

$$\frac{\textit{Autopsies performed on intermediate and late fetal deaths for a period} \times 100}{\textit{Total intermediate and late fetal deaths for the same period}}$$

Example: A hospital newborn service reported 12 fetal deaths last quarter: 6 early, 4 intermediate, and 2 late. Of these, the two late fetal deaths and one intermediate fetal death were autopsied. Applying the formula above, the fetal autopsy rate for this hospital is 50.00 percent.

$$\frac{((2 \textit{ late fetal death autopsies} + 1 \textit{ intermediate fetal death autopsy}) \times 100)}{(4+2)} = 50.00\%$$

Exercise 7.11

Using the information in the table below, calculate (round to two decimal places) the newborn death, fetal death, newborn autopsy, and fetal autopsy rates for the Newborn Service at University Hospital. In this exercise, the newborn deaths are included in the newborn discharges.

University Hospital
Newborn Service Statistics
January–June 20XX

Births	622
Discharges	620
Newborn deaths	3
Newborn Autopsies	1
Fetal Deaths	
Early	6
Intermediate	4
Late	2
Fetal Death Autopsies	
Early	1
Intermediate	1
Late	1

Answers:

Newborn death rate:

Fetal death rate:

Newborn autopsy rate:

Fetal autopsy rate:

Exercise 7.12

Community Healthcare System reported the statistics in the table below for its four facilities during its past semiannual period. Calculate (round to two decimal places) the newborn death, fetal death, newborn autopsy, and fetal autopsy rates for each facility and for the system as a whole. In this exercise, the deaths are included in the discharges.

Community Healthcare System
Newborn Statistics
July–December 20XX

	Urban Hospital	Suburban Hospital	Rural Hospital	Specialty Hospital
Live Births	240	235	165	198
Newborn discharges	239	230	162	195
Newborn Deaths	2	1	2	16
Fetal deaths:				
Early	5	2	1	7
Intermediate	3	3	1	6
Late	2	1	1	5
Autopsies				
Newborn	1	0	1	6
Fetal (late and intermediate)	2	1	2	7

Answers:

Urban Hospital
Newborn death rate:

Fetal death rate:

Newborn autopsy rate:

Fetal autopsy rate:

(continued on next page)

Exercise 7.12 (continued)

Suburban Hospital
Newborn death rate:

Fetal death rate:

Newborn autopsy rate:

Fetal autopsy rate:

Rural Hospital
Newborn death rate:

Fetal death rate:

Newborn autopsy rate:

Fetal autopsy rate:

Specialty Hospital
Newborn death rate:

Fetal death rate:

Newborn autopsy rate:

Fetal autopsy rate:

Chapter 7 Test

(Calculate all rates to two decimal places)

Community Hospital reported the statistics in the table below. Using these data, calculate the rates requested below and select the correct calculation for each.

Community Hospital
Annual Statistics 20XX

Inpatient discharges	
Adults and children	7,356
Newborn	730
Inpatient deaths: (included in discharges)	
Adults and children	60
Newborn	2
Fetal deaths:	
Early	6
Intermediate	3
Late	2
Inpatient autopsies:	
Adults and children	12
Newborn	2
Coroner's cases	
Unavailable for autopsy	3
Autopsy by hospital pathologist (included in inpatient autopsies)	1
Fetal death autopsies:	
Intermediate and late	3
Former hospital patient brought in for autopsy	1

1. Gross autopsy rate

    a. 22.00%
    b. 22.58%
    c. 0.22%
    d. 2.25%

2. Net autopsy rate

    a. 23.73%
    b. 22.58%
    c. 2.37%
    d. 0.23%

(continued on next page)

Chapter 7 Test (continued)

3. Adjusted hospital autopsy rate

    a. 23.73%
    b. 23.81%
    c. 25.00%
    d. 0.23%

4. What is the newborn autopsy rate?

5. What is the fetal death autopsy rate?

Using the data reported by University Hospital for June 20XX in the table below, calculate the rates (round to two decimal places).

University Hospital
June 20XX
Statistics

Discharges	
Total adults and children	1,166
Newborn	132
Total live births	135
Deaths: (included in discharges)	
Adults and children	198
Newborn	5
Autopsies:	
Adults and children	20
Newborn	4
Hospital autopsied outpatients	7
Coroner's cases (unavailable for autopsy)	3
Fetal deaths:	
Early	2
Intermediate	3
Late	2
Fetal death autopsies:	
Intermediate and late	3

6. Gross death rate

7. Gross autopsy rate

8. Net autopsy rate

Chapter 7 Test (continued)

9. Adjusted hospital autopsy rate

10. Newborn autopsy rate

11. Fetal death rate

12. Fetal autopsy rate

13. Using the data in the table below, calculate the gross death, gross autopsy, and net autopsy rates for each month and the year for University Hospital.

University Hospital
Annual Statistics
20XX

Month	Discharges	Inpatient Deaths	Autopsies	Coroner's Cases	Gross Death Rate	Gross Autopsy Rate	Net Autopsy Rate
January	601	5	1	1			
February	585	5	1	2			
March	620	8	6	1			
April	660	2	1	0			
May	621	6	2	1			
June	612	6	3	2			
July	592	9	5	3			
August	589	3	2	0			
September	587	5	2	1			
October	601	6	3	1			
November	611	3	1	0			
December	585	2	1	1			
Totals							

(continued on next page)

Chapter 7 Test (continued)

14. Which of the following represents a hospital autopsy? List as many letters as apply.

    a. A former inpatient died at home a month after discharge from the hospital, and his body was brought to the hospital for autopsy.

    b. The coroner authorized the hospital pathologist to perform an autopsy on a patient who died in the ESD after a car accident.

    c. A patient who had been receiving radiation therapy on an outpatient basis at the hospital died at home; her body was brought to the hospital for autopsy.

    d. A victim of gunshot wounds who died in the ESD was autopsied by the medical examiner.

    e. A cardiac patient died in the ESD, and the hospital pathologist performed the autopsy.

    f. The hospital pathologist designated a physician to cover for her while she was away. The physician performed an autopsy on a deceased hospital inpatient.

    g. A late fetal death (stillbirth) was autopsied by the hospital pathologist.

15. What is the principal difference between net autopsy rate and adjusted hospital autopsy rate?

    a. Fetal deaths are not counted in hospital autopsy rates.

    b. Hospital autopsy rates include only those deaths where the bodies are available for autopsy.

    c. The net autopsy rate considers only inpatient deaths.

    d. Legal cases sometimes are excluded from deaths when computing net autopsy rate.

16. The hospital pathologist or some other designated physician is generally the individual allowed to perform autopsies. True or False?

17. In which of the following rates are outpatients who were autopsied counted in an autopsy rate?

    a. Gross autopsy rate

    b. Net autopsy rate

    c. Adjusted hospital autopsy rate

    d. Newborn autopsy rate

18. Why are fetal deaths never counted in any autopsy rate except the fetal autopsy rate?

Chapter 7 Test (continued)

Indicate whether the statements below are true or false. If an answer is false, explain why.

19. To be considered a hospital autopsy, an autopsy must be performed by the staff pathologist or a physician delegated the responsibility.

20. A hospital autopsy must be performed in the hospital.

21. Hospital autopsies are performed only on inpatients.

22. Autopsies on fetuses are included in hospital autopsies.

23. The essentials of a hospital autopsy are that it be performed by the hospital pathologist or a physician delegated the responsibility, there is a consent from the patient's next of kin or legal representative, that an autopsy report be filed in the patient's health record, and that tissue specimens and the autopsy report be filed in the hospital laboratory.

24. The net autopsy rate includes both inpatients and out-of-hospital patients.

25. A deceased hospital inpatient whose body is released to legal authorities for autopsy is not included in the computation of the net autopsy rate.

Chapter 8
Morbidity and Other Miscellaneous Rates

Objectives

At the conclusion of this chapter, you should be able to:

- Define nosocomial infection
- Discuss and calculate infection rate
- Define and calculate the postoperative infection rate
- Distinguish between a surgical procedure and a surgical operation
- When provided with appropriate data, compute the following rates: C-section, consultation, and other rates

Infection Rate

The term **morbidity** means the state of being diseased or the number of sick persons or cases of disease in relation to a specific population. Morbidity may be infectious or have other causes. For example, the presence of **concomitant** (taking place at the same time), **chronic** (of long duration) conditions may constitute comorbidity. Moreover, morbidity may be preexisting (occurring prior to admission to the hospital) or **iatrogenic** (occurring because of the patient's treatment).

Preventing morbidity due to infection is an important quality management function. Frequently, the healthcare facility establishes a committee whose primary function is to evaluate infections and determine their causes so that recurrence can be avoided. Typically called the infection control committee, it is composed of representatives from medical staff, nursing, pharmacy, risk management, and health information management. Charged with the duty of infection control, committee members establish procedures for the management and reporting of infections. Effective management of infections acquired in the hospital (**nosocomial infections**) sometimes requires finding cases beyond the infections listed by physicians in the medical record. The HIM practitioner can help identify such cases in the course of performing qualitative analysis and/or coding.

In 1970, the CDC developed The National Nosocomial Infections Surveillance (NNIS) System to monitor the incidence of nosocomial infections. They are referred to as healthcare-associated infections (HAIs). This is a voluntary reporting system and is the only national system for tracking nosocomial infections (CDC 2005).

As defined in chapter 2, the term *rate* refers to the number of times something happened compared to the number of times it could have happened (Rate = Part/Base or R = P/B). Each healthcare facility's medical staff must determine the criteria for inclusion of a patient in both the numerator (infection) and denominator (patients at risk of infection).

Most healthcare facilities differentiate between nosocomial infections and exacerbation and recurrence of previous infections. For example, if an obstetrical patient develops a urinary tract infection, a physician must determine whether it was hospital acquired or due to a recurrence of a previous urinary tract infection. In addition, the infection control committee determines whether nosocomial infections are attributable to specific patient care units (PCUs), specific operations, patients with specified diseases, the organized medical staff units, or individual physicians or hospital employees.

The nosocomial infection rate is the number of hospital-acquired infections in the hospital for a given time period divided by the total number of inpatient discharges (including deaths) for the same time period.

The formula for calculating the nosocomial infection rate is:

$$\frac{Total\ number\ of\ nosocomial\ infections\ for\ a\ period \times 100}{Total\ number\ of\ discharges,\ including\ deaths,\ for\ the\ same\ period}$$

Example: In January, Community Hospital had 350 discharges and deaths. Thirteen of these patients had hospital-acquired infections. The nosocomial infection rate is 3.7%.

$$\frac{(13 \times 100)}{350} = 3.7\%$$

Infection rates may be calculated separately for specific infections such as surgical wound infections, puerperal infections (infections that occur immediately after childbirth), and infections of the respiratory tract, urinary tract, bloodstream, and so on.

The formula for calculating the infection rate is:

$$\frac{Total\ number\ of\ infections \times 100}{Total\ number\ of\ discharges\ (including\ deaths)\ for\ the\ period}$$

Example: In July, Community Hospital had 150 discharges, eight of whom developed a urinary tract infection while in the hospital. The infection rate is calculated by placing the number of infections (8) × 100 in the numerator and dividing by the 150 (discharges) in the denominator.

$$\frac{(8 \times 100)}{150} = 5.33\%$$

In addition to infections, healthcare facilities are concerned with any other type of complication that results from, or occurs during, the course of care. Other types of complications that require special attention by medical staff and administration include wound disruptions, decubitus ulcers, postoperative hemorrhages, and adverse drug reactions.

Example: In August, Community Hospital had 12 patients on the Medicine unit who had a blood transfusion, of those, two developed an adverse reaction to the transfusion. The blood transfusion reaction rate is calculated by placing the number of blood transfusion reactions (2) × 100 in the numerator and dividing it by the number of blood transfusions.

$$\frac{(2 \times 100)}{12} = 16.67\%$$

Exercise 8.1

Based on the information in the table below, calculate (round to two decimal places) the rates requested for Community Hospital. In this exercise deaths are included in the discharges.

Community Hospital
Annual Statistics
20XX

Discharges:	
Adults and children	1,784
Newborn	123
Deaths:	
Adults and children	12
Newborn	1
Nosocomial infections:	
Adults and children	13
Newborn	3

1. Nosocomial infection rate for adults and children

2. Nosocomial infection rate for newborns

3. Total nosocomial infection rate for the hospital

4. Gross death rate for this annual period

Answers:

Nosocomial infection rate for adults and children:

Nosocomial infection rate for newborns:

Total nosocomial infection rate for the hospital:

Gross death rate for this annual period:

Exercise 8.2

Based on the information given in the table below, calculate (round to two decimal places) the rates requested. In this exercise the deaths are included in the discharges.

**University Hospital
Semiannual Statistics
January–June 20XX**

Service	No. Discharges	No. of Deaths	No. of Nosocomial Infections
Medicine	2,333	212	28
Surgery	2,532	102	32
Obstetrics	623	2	3
Psychiatry	452	1	3
Rehabilitation	987	14	19
Pediatrics	832	1	2
Newborn	625	0	2
Totals			

1. Gross death rate for each service

2. Total gross death rate

3. Nosocomial infection rate for each service

4. Nosocomial infection rate for the semiannual period

Answers:

Gross death rate for each service:

Total gross death rate:

Nosocomial infection rate for each service:

Nosocomial infection rate for the semiannual period:

Postoperative Infection Rate

Another specific type of infection of great concern to hospitals is the **postoperative infection rate**. This is because a postoperative infection can contribute to the increased morbidity, mortality, and cost of care. Postoperative infections occur, as the name suggests, after surgery. Even though hospitals take care to avoid an infection after surgery, one still can occur.

Two terms need to be considered here:

- A *surgical procedure* is defined as any single, separate, systematic process upon or within the body that can be complete in itself; normally is performed by a physician, dentist, or other licensed practitioner; can be performed with or without instruments; and is performed to restore disunited or deficient parts, remove diseased or injured tissues, extract foreign matter, assist in obstetrical delivery, or aid in diagnosis.

- A *surgical operation* is defined as one or more surgical procedures performed at one time for one patient via a common approach or for a common purpose.

  — An example of a surgical operation including more than one surgical procedure is an abdominoperitoneal resection, which involves resection of both the abdomen and the peritoneum.

  — An example of two surgical operations and two surgical procedures is a tonsillectomy followed by a circumcision. Even though the procedures were performed at one time for one patient, the approach to each procedure is different and the two procedures are not performed for a common purpose.

The postoperative infection rate is the ratio of all infections in clean surgical cases to the number of surgical operations performed. A general definition of a **clean surgical case** is one in which no infection existed prior to surgery.

The formula for calculating the postoperative infection rate is:

$$\frac{Total\ number\ of\ infections\ in\ clean\ surgical\ cases\ for\ a\ period \times 100}{Number\ of\ surgical\ operations\ for\ the\ period}$$

Example: During November, a hospital reported that 758 surgical operations were performed. The infection control committee reported one postoperative infection in a clean surgical case. According to the formula, the postoperative infection rate for November is 0.13 percent.

$$\frac{(1 \times 100)}{758} = \frac{100}{758} = 0.1319 = 0.13\%$$

A postoperative infection may be difficult to determine because it is not always evident whether the patient entered the hospital with an infection or acquired one because of the surgical techniques used. Therefore, the medical staff should provide guidance to the HIM practitioner and the Infection Control Department on what constitutes a clean surgical case and which infections should be considered postoperative infections.

Many Infection Control Departments use the classifications developed by the National Nosocomial Infections Surveillance System. These are developed according to the likelihood and degree of wound contamination at the time of the operation. Wounds are classified as clean, clean-contaminated, contaminated, and dirty or infected wounds.

Their descriptions include a clean wound as one in which no inflammation is encountered and the respiratory, alimentary, genital, or uninfected urinary tracts are not entered. Many Infection Control Departments report the number of postoperative infections relative to the type of surgery that was performed. For example, if a patient has no infection prior to a coronary artery bypass graft, but develops one after surgery, then the Infection Control Department would report this as a postoperative infection in a clean case.

A clean-contaminated case is one in which the respiratory, alimentary, genital, or urinary tract is entered. Specifically, operations involving the biliary tract, appendix, vagina, and oropharynx are included in this category. For instance, a patient that develops an infection after an abdominal hysterectomy would be reported as an infection in a clean-contaminated case.

A contaminated wound includes an open, fresh, accidental wound; an operation with a break in sterile technique or gross spillage from the gastrointestinal tract and incisions in which acute, nonpurulent inflammation is encountered.

A dirty wound is one that involves existing clinical infection or perforated viscera.

If you are assisting the Infection Control Department with their statistics, be sure to determine how they are classifying your facility's postoperative infections.

Exercise 8.3

Based on the information in the table below, calculate (round to two decimal places) the postoperative infection and postoperative death rates for University Hospital during this semiannual period

University Hospital
Surgery Service
July–December 20XX

Number of surgical operations	2,059
Number of patients operated on	2,053
Number of postoperative infections	12
Number of postoperative deaths	10

Answers:

Postoperative infection rate:

Postoperative death rate:

Exercise 8.4

Based on the information in the table below, calculate (round to two decimal places) the rates requested below.

**University Hospital
Surgery Service
July–December 20XX Statistics**

Month	Disch*	Deaths Postop	Other	Infections Postop	Nosocomial	No. of Patients Operated	No. of Surgical Operations
Jul	620	3	12	3	5	301	302
Aug	560	2	10	2	4	293	299
Sep	600	2	9	3	3	312	315
Oct	558	4	11	3	4	299	302
Nov	690	3	14	2	3	306	306
Dec	682	4	14	3	2	314	316
Total							

*Deaths are included.

Answers:

1. The month with the lowest postoperative infection rate:

2. The postoperative infection rate for the semiannual period:

3. The month with the highest postoperative death rate:

4. The postoperative death rate for the semiannual period:

5. The gross death rate for the surgical service during the semiannual period:

Cesarean-Section Rate

Most hospitals determine the percentage of deliveries that are performed by Cesarean section (commonly called C-section) as compared to spontaneous or vaginal deliveries. Much attention has been given to high C-section rates by specific physicians, hospitals, and areas of the country because of concerns about adverse effects to the mother and child. Additionally, it may be necessary to report C-section rates to accrediting agencies or the American Medical Association (AMA) for such reasons as residency programs.

A **delivery** is defined as the process of delivering a liveborn infant or dead fetus (and placenta) by manual, instrumental, or surgical means.

Handy Tip: A pregnant mother who delivers has one delivery but may have multiple births. For example, a woman who delivers a liveborn infant is counted as one delivery and one live birth whereas a woman who delivers liveborn twins is counted as one delivery and two live births. A woman who delivers a stillbirth is counted as one delivery and one intermediate or late fetal death. This is also considered to be one delivery and one birth since a stillbirth is considered to be a birth, but not a live birth.

Sometimes a woman is admitted to the hospital for a condition of her pregnancy but does not deliver her infant during that hospitalization. For example, a woman may be admitted in apparent labor, which turns out to be false labor. In this case, the patient may be classified as an obstetrics patient, not delivered.

The formula for calculating the Cesarean-section rate is:

$$\frac{Total\ number\ of\ C\text{-}sections\ performed\ in\ a\ period \times 100}{Total\ number\ of\ deliveries\ in\ the\ period\ (including\ C\text{-}sections)}$$

Handy Tip: The C-section rate is not based on the number of patients discharged but, rather, on the number of deliveries. A rate compares the number of actual occurrences with the total possible; obviously, only deliveries can be C-sections. Usually the data on deliveries and the number of C-sections for the period are obtained from delivery room personnel. First-time C-sections are often reported to the medical staff by either the delivery room personnel or the HIM practitioner.

Example: Three C-sections were performed in a month during which there were 360 deliveries. The C-section rate is calculated by multiplying the number of C-sections (3) by 100 and then dividing that number by the total number of deliveries (360). The C-section rate is 0.83 percent.

$$\frac{(3 \times 100)}{360} = \frac{300}{360} = 0.83\%$$

Exercise 8.5

Based on the information in the table below, calculate (round to two decimal places) the C-section rate at University Hospital for the semiannual period.

University Hospital
Obstetrics Service
Semiannual Statistics
January–June 20XX

Admissions	526
Discharges:	
Delivered	394
Not delivered	120
Aborted	12
Vaginal deliveries	316
C-sections	78

Answer:

C-section rate:

Exercise 8.6

Based on the information in the table below, calculate (round to two decimal places) the C-section rate, the newborn death rate, and the fetal death rate at University Hospital for the month of May.

University Hospital
Newborn Service
May 20XX

Discharges (includes deaths)	150
Births:	
Single live births	138
Multiple live births	1 set of twins
	1 set of triplets
Deliveries:	
Vaginal	119
C-section	27

Exercise 8.6 (continued)

Deaths:

Newborn	1
Fetal:	
Early	4
Intermediate	3
Late	3

Answers:

C-section rate:

Newborn death rate:

Fetal death rate:

Consultation Rates

A **consultation** is the response by one healthcare professional to another healthcare professional's request to provide recommendations and/or opinions regarding the care of a particular patient/resident. A patient's attending physician may occasionally request that a consultant (another physician or healthcare practitioner) examine a patient and give an opinion as to his or her condition. The consultant also should review the medical record and then prepare a consultation report that includes the findings of the examination and recommendations for treating the patient.

The formula for calculating the consultation rate is:

$$\frac{Total\ number\ of\ patients\ receiving\ a\ consultation \times 100}{Total\ number\ of\ patients\ discharged}$$

Handy Tip: Close examination of this formula reveals that the definition of a rate applies here. That is, every patient discharged could theoretically have had a consultation.

Example: During the past month, a medicine unit had 93 discharges, 12 of whom were seen by a consultant. The consultation rate is 12.9 percent.

$$\frac{(12 \times 100)}{93} = \frac{1,200}{93} = 12.90\%$$

Exercise 8.7

Based on the information in the table below, calculate the consultation rate (round to two decimal places) at Community Hospital for each service and the total for the semiannual period.

Community Hospital
Semiannual Statistics
January–June, 20XX

Service	Discharges	No. of Patients Receiving Consultations	Consultation Rate
Medicine	2,880	864	
Surgery	2,160	701	
Obstetrics	685	26	
Psychiatric	142	6	
Rehabilitation	156	12	
Pediatrics	251	42	
Newborn	672	2	
Totals			

Exercise 8.8

Based on the information in the table below, calculate (round to two decimal places) the rates requested below for Community Hospital. In this exercise, the deaths are included in the discharges.

Community Hospital
Surgery Service
Annual Statistics 20XX

Month	Discharges	Deaths	Consultations	Consultation Rate	Gross Death Rate
January	576	17	115		
February	589	12	102		
March	601	15	84		
April	542	13	63		
May	614	6	96		
June	574	14	85		
July	563	10	74		
August	555	9	69		
September	603	6	78		
October	591	7	45		
November	583	5	86		
December	562	12	73		
Totals					

1. Consultation rate for each month:

2. Consultation rate for the year for the surgery service:

3. Gross death rate for each month:

4. Gross death rate for the year for the surgery service:

Other Rates

The HIM practitioner may compute and report other rates according to individual healthcare facility needs. External agencies may also ask that additional data and rates be reported. To pursue all the possibilities in this book is impractical. The best rule of thumb is to use the "other rates" formula. You may become so intrigued with this formula that you will volunteer to produce new and useful rates, which is, incidentally, part of the HIM professional's responsibility. The formula for calculating other rates is:

$$\frac{Number\ of\ times\ something\ happened \times 100}{Number\ of\ times\ something\ could\ have\ happened}$$

Handy Tip: Statistics should not be kept just because they have always been kept. After you assure yourself, the administration, and the medical staff that a particular statistic no longer serves a useful purpose, stop keeping it. Do not be afraid to be creative and imaginative about providing new ideas for statistical computations that will serve a useful purpose, even if only on a temporary, special-study basis.

Exercise 8.9

Based on the information in the table below, calculate (round to two decimal places) the readmission rates requested below for University Hospital, using the following formula:

$$\frac{Number\ of\ patients\ readmitted\ within\ 30\ days\ of\ the\ previous\ discharge \times 100}{Total\ patients\ discharged\ (including\ deaths)}$$

University Hospital
Surgery Service
Semiannual Statistics
January–June 20XX

Month	Discharges	No. of Patients Readmitted Within 30 days of the Previous Discharge	Readmission Rate
January	562	27	
February	654	32	
March	678	38	
April	649	21	
May	658	25	
June	667	34	
Totals			

1. The readmission rate for each month:

2. The total readmission rate for the period:

Exercise 8.10

Based on the information in the table below, calculate (round to two decimal places) the rate of nondelivered patients and aborted patients at University Hospital for each month and for the quarter.

University Hospital
Obstetrics Department
Fourth Quarter Statistics 20XX

Month	No. of Patients Delivered	No. of Patients Not Delivered	No. of Patients who Aborted	Nondelivered Rate	Abortion Rate
October	402	12	6		
November	385	20	5		
December	391	18	3		
Totals					

Exercise 8.11

Based on the information in the table below for University Hospital, calculate (round to two decimal places) the rate of accounts turned over to collection for each month and for the period. Use the formula for a rate to answer this question.

University Hospital
Semiannual Statistics
July–December 20XX

Month	No. of Discharges	No. of Accounts Turned over to a Collection Agency	Rate of Accounts Turned over to a Collection Agency
July	302	25	
August	326	30	
September	342	32	
October	318	15	
November	352	24	
December	312	19	
Totals			

Exercise 8.12

Based on the information in the table below for Community Hospital, calculate (round to two decimal places) the complication rate for each service and the total for this semiannual period.

**Community Hospital
Statistics
July–December 20XX**

Service	Discharges	Complications	Complication Rate
Medicine	1,742	142	
Surgery	1,080	180	
Obstetrics	389	3	
Newborn	390	1	
Total			

Exercise 8.13

Based on the information in the table below, calculate (round to two decimal places) the rates requested below.

**Community Hospital
Medicine Service
Selected Annual Statistics 20XX**

Total Hospital Discharges 7,201

Medicine Service	Number
Discharges	4,523
Complications	125
Nosocomial infections	78
Deaths (included in discharges)	60
Payer information:	
Medicare	905
Medicaid	812
Third party insurance	2,126
Self-pay	680

Exercise 8.13 (continued)

Selected patients:

Primary diagnosis:

Cancer	986
Diabetes and its complications	625
HIV/AIDS	123
Myocardial infarction	450
Asthma	267
Substance abuse	98

Answers:

Percentage of patients in the Medicine service:

Complication rate:

Nosocomial infection rate:

Medicine service gross death rate:

Percentage of patients with:
Medicare:

Medicaid:

Third party insurance:

Self-pay:

(continued on next page)

Exercise 8.13 (continued)

Percentage of patients with:
Cancer:

Diabetes and its complications:

HIV/AIDS:

Myocardial infarction:

Asthma:

Substance abuse:

Chapter 8 Test

Indicate whether the following statements are true or false.

1. Every healthcare facility must keep infection rates for each of its medical care units.

2. A nosocomial infection is an infection that was acquired while a patient was hospitalized.

3. The postoperative infection rate is the ratio of all infections in clean surgical cases to the number of surgical procedures.

4. A patient who has a salpingo-oophorectomy would be counted as having one surgical procedure and one surgical operation.

5. A patient who had a colonoscopy and removal of two moles on his neck at the same time would be counted as having one surgical operation and two procedures.

Chapter 8 Test (continued)

Complete statements 6 and 7 below using the annual statistics reported in the table below.

Discharges:	
Adults and children	7,280
Newborn	798
Surgical procedures	1,265
Surgical operations	1,260
Patients receiving consultations	1,999
Nosocomial infections	23

6. The hospital infection rate (including newborns) is:

   a. 0.02%
   b. 0.28%
   c. 2.80%
   d. 28.00%

7. The consultation rate (including newborns) is:

   a. 0.02%
   b. 0.24%
   c. 2.75%
   d. 24.75%

8. A hospital reports the following statistics for the past year: births, 1,345; deliveries, 1,340; C-sections, 60; and obstetrical discharges, 1,425. The C-section rate for that year is:

   a. 0.47%
   b. 1.47%
   c. 4.48%
   d. 44.78%

9. A women's hospital reported 212 deliveries during June. Two sets of twins were born. There were 215 obstetrical discharges; 214 births; four women had first-time C-sections; and three women had a repeat C-section. The C-section rate for June is 3.30 percent. True or False?

10. What is the percentage of multiple births?

   a. 0.93%
   b. 93.5%
   c. 1.87%
   d. 0.94%

(continued on next page)

Chapter 8 Test (continued)

11. What is the percentage of patients with multiple births?
    a. 0.93%
    b. 0.94%
    c. 94.0%
    d. 0.65%

12. A third-party review company reported the statistics in the table below. Calculate (round to two decimal places) the rate of admissions approved for each month and for the quarter.

	July	August	September
Number of customers	412	4,415	419
Number of admission claims reviewed	927	935	956
Number of claims approved for admission to the hospital	912	927	931

Answers:

July:

August:

September:

Chapter 9

Statistics Computed within the Health Information Management Department

Objectives

At the conclusion of this chapter, you should be able to:

- Describe the uses of statistics computed within the HIM department in terms of unit cost, productivity, and staffing levels

- Recognize how statistics are used in the creation of the health information department budget

- Define budget and differentiate between the operational and capital budgets

- Verify computerized statistical reports for accuracy

- Recalculate statistics for greater specificity

- Generate computerized statistical reports

Health Information Statistics

Statistics computed for use within the health information management (HIM) department usually relate to labor costs, productivity, and staffing, and often are used in determining whether the department may be able to hire a new employee, setting benchmarks for productivity, determining absentee rates, and so on. The following sections provide examples of common, everyday computations made by HIM staff members.

Employee Compensation and Unit Labor Costs

One example of where health information managers must make effective decisions is in regard to employee compensation and **unit labor cost**.

The annual compensation for an individual employee is calculated by multiplying the number of hours worked per year (2,080 for a full-time employee) by the hourly wage and then multiplying that number by the benefits received. A sample calculation would be:

2,080 hours × $10 per hour × 30% benefits = $20,800 + .30 = $6,240 + $20,800 = $27,040

Handy Tip: A quicker way to compute this is to multiply by 1.3 (if 30% benefits).

2,080 hours × $10 per hour × 1.3 (30% benefits) = $27,040

To determine the annual productivity, multiply the amount of work completed (for example, lines transcribed, number of records coded and the like) per day by the number of workdays in the year (5 workdays per week × 52 weeks per year = 260 workdays). Note that this calculation includes any vacation time or sick leave that an employee may take.

The unit labor cost is determined by dividing the total annual compensation by total annual productivity. For example, workload in a transcription section of a department is commonly measured in lines or minutes of dictation transcribed by the staff. To determine the unit transcription labor cost, divide the total transcriptionist annual compensation by the total annual productivity as shown below.

$$\frac{Total \ (sum) \ medical \ transcriptionist \ annual \ compensation}{Total \ (sum) \ medical \ transcriptionist \ annual \ productivity}$$

Example: Two full-time transcriptionists in the HIM department produce 1,000 lines each per day. One employee earns $12.00 per hour and is paid an annual salary of $24,960; the other employee earns $15.00 per hour and is paid an annual salary of $31,200.

To determine the annual productivity, multiply the number of lines transcribed by the two employees (1,000 per day per transcriptionist or 2,000 per day) by the number of workdays in the year (5 workdays per week × 52 weeks per year = 260 workdays).

2(260 workdays × 1,000 lines) = 520,000 lines per year

To determine the unit cost, add the two salaries ($24,960 + $31,200 = $56,160) and divide by the total number of lines transcribed by the two employees in one year (520,000). The unit cost is $0.108 or 11 cents per line.

$$\frac{\$56,160}{520,000} = \$0.108 = \$0.11$$

Example: This formula can be applied to other employees in the department. For example, one coder is compensated at $12.00 per hour and codes six records per hour. The employee's annual compensation is $24,960.

To determine the employee's annual productivity, multiply six records per hour by 7.5 hours per day to get 45 records per day. Then multiply 45 by 5 days in the workweek and 52 weeks in the year to get 11,700 records coded per year. The unit cost is $2.13 per record.

Handy Tip: Some employers consider 7.5 hours a productive work day, thinking in terms of 8-hour day minus breaks the employee may take.

Handy Tip: Notice that the unit cost did not consider times that the employee is not working (for example, sick time or vacation time). The unit cost to code one record is still valid because someone has to perform the work even when the employee who normally performs that task is absent.

Exercise 9.1

Complete the exercises below.

1. Transcriptionist A is a full-time employee earning $13.00 per hour and an annual salary of $27,040. She transcribes 1,200 lines per day for a total of 312,000 lines per year. What is the unit medical transcription labor cost for transcriptionist A (or, how much does a line cost when transcribed by transcriptionist A)?

2. Transcriptionist B is a full-time employee earning $10.00 per hour and an annual salary of $20,800. He transcribes 900 lines per day for a total of 234,000 lines per year. What is the unit medical transcription labor cost for transcriptionist B?

3. A HIM department has eight full-time transcriptionists. Five of them produce 1,000 lines each per day. Of these five, one earns $12.00 per hour, three earn $12.50 per hour, and one earns $13.00 per hour.

   Two other transcriptionists in the department produce 1,100 lines per day. Of these two, one earns $13.00 per hour and the other earns $14.00 per hour. Finally, the eighth transcriptionist produces 1,200 lines per day and earns $12.00 per hour.

   a. What is the difference in cost per line between the employee who produces 1,000 lines per day and makes $12.00 per hour and the employee who produces 1,200 lines per day and makes $12.00 per hour?
   b. What general observations can you make about the unit labor cost and the two employees just mentioned?

(continued on next page)

Exercise 9.1 (continued)

c. What is the difference in cost per line between the employee who produces 1,000 lines per day and makes $13.00 per hour and the employee who produces 1,100 lines per day and makes $13.00 per hour?

d. What is the total unit cost for medical transcription?

To justify costs for releases of information (ROI) in the health information department, one HIM professional needed to calculate cost breakdowns. (See table 9.1.)

The Health Information Portability and Accountability Act (HIPAA), commonly referred to as the Privacy Rule, allows a facility to charge a reasonable, cost-based fee for any requests for records made by patients after the first request. The first request each year must be made without charge to the patient. Time studies would need to be performed in order to validate the cost. This may involve:

- Keeping track of the time it takes to review the request and log it into your computer system

- Finding the patient information in the master patient index

- Determining the location of the medical record, either paper or electronic

Table 9.1.   Average Record Requests per Month

Community Hospital Health Information Department Release of Information Costs Average Requests per month = 360	
Item	**Cost per request**
Postage: $305 per month	$\frac{\$305}{360} = 0.847 = \$0.85$
Service contract (includes copier): $100 per month	$\frac{\$100}{360} = 0.277 = \$0.28$
Equipment (includes copies): $125 per month	$\frac{\$125}{360} = 0.347 = \$0.35$
Supplies (includes toner, printer cartridges, paper): $75 per month	$\frac{\$75}{360} = 0.208 = \$0.21$
Wages: $12.00 per hour = monthly salary of $2,080 ($12.00 \times 2080$ hours $= \$24,960; \frac{\$24,960}{12} = \$2,080$)	$\frac{\$2,080}{360} = 5.777 = \$5.78$
Total	**$7.47**

- Determining whether other departments have portions of the medical record and have possibly made a disclosure

- Retrieving the record if it is a paper record or locating the record online and printing any scanned documents

- Reviewing any previous disclosures made

- Preparing a list of the disclosures

- Preparing an invoice for the patient

- Updating the release of information log

The HIM department also may consider nonlabor expenses such as those listed in table 9.1. However, the facility's chief financial officer is usually consulted to determine whether other nonlabor costs can be applied.

Exercise 9.2

Using the information in the table below, calculate the cost breakdown per item and the monthly cost for the release of information (ROI) services at Community Hospital.

Community Hospital
Health Information Department
Release of Information Costs
Average Requests per month = 482

Item	Cost per month
Postage	$365
Service contract (includes copier)	$85
Equipment (includes copies)	$122
Supplies (includes toner, printer cartridges, paper)	$92
Wages	$11.50 per hour
Monthly cost	

Exercise 9.3

Using the information provided in the table below, complete the following exercises.

Community Hospital
Health Information Department
Release of Information Costs
Average Requests per month = 542

Item	Cost per month
Postage	$456
Service contract (includes copier)	$216
Equipment (includes copies)	$135
Supplies (includes toner, printer cartridges, paper)	$110
Wages	$11.00 per hour

1. Calculate the cost breakdown for each item.

2. What is the monthly cost for the ROI services?

3. On average, the ROI section brings in $1,800 per month. What is the difference between cost and income?

Other Labor Unit Costs

The HIM department also processes patient record (chart) requests, which consumes a great deal of staff time. Responsibilities in maintaining records include:

- *Chart pulls*: Even as the need to pull records of previous patients diminishes with the use of an **electronic health record** (EHR), the HIM department will still need to determine costs and productivity standards for this position. A combination of paper and electronic records will continue to be in use for some time, and both manual and electronic processes will be used to maintain the record. This combination is referred to as a **hybrid health record**. The types of statistics may include the number of requests for the paper record versus electronic records or the number needed as stat (immediately) versus routine requests.

- *Scanning of records*: Some facilities choose to scan the paper record to make it available online. These facilities may have an electronic document management system (EDMS) to help manage all their documents for a patient. This new technology allows users to scan documents, move documents from the transcription system to the EHR, enter information online, handle the **electronic signature** of records, index documents as they are entered into the computer system, and access information from a variety of locations, to name a few functions. This will necessitate the types of statistics desired to determine who is using the system, how the electronic signature is given, where providers are signing, and so forth. New technologies will continue to evolve, and managers in health information departments will continue to determine the costs and benefits of these new systems.

- *Provider–patient e-mail*: As patients become more comfortable with e-mailing their physicians and as healthcare insurers begin to reimburse physicians for their time used to e-mail patients, this will become an everyday issue for healthcare organizations. E-mail and text messages are considered to be healthcare business records and thus are subject to the same rules and regulations as any other health record. E-mail can be used to schedule appointments, refill prescriptions, or transfer department results. Organizations may decide to keep track of the time spent responding to e-mails, gathering information before the e-mail is answered, and deciding what can be answered via e-mail.

- *Loose papers*: The number of pieces of paper received in the HIM department for filing is a significant factor in determining staffing levels. Loose papers may be measured in inches or by individual pieces, which is a more accurate measure. Because of the time involved in tracking this information, departments may choose to sample this activity for a one-week period several times a year.

Exercise 9.4

Complete the following two exercises.

1. The HIM department at Community Hospital completed a time study, and the data are listed in the table below. Complete the table by determining the number of hours worked in each activity.

Community Hospital
Health Information Department
Time Allocation Report
September 20XX

Service/Division	Number of hours	Hours Worked
Inpatient records:		
Pediatrics	11.75 h/w x 4 weeks	
Obstetrics	59.5 h/w x 4 weeks	
Psychiatric	98.5 h/w x 4 weeks	
Newborn	50.75 h/w x 4 weeks	
Medicine	426.75 h/w x 4 weeks	
Surgery	447 h/w x 4 weeks	
Subtotal inpatient records		
ED Records:		
Clerical/Processing	28 h/w x 4 weeks	
Correspondence	7 h/w x 4 weeks	
Supervisory	5 h/w x 4 weeks	
Subtotal ED records		
General clinic:		
Clerical/processing	6 h/w x 4 weeks	
Supervisory	0.5 h/w x 4 weeks	
Transcription	0.10 h/record x 170 records	
Subtotal general clinic		

Exercise 9.4 (continued)

Outpatient/ambulatory surgery

Clerical/primary:	21.5 h/w x 4 weeks
Filing	5.25 h/w x 4 weeks
Admissions	2.5 h/w x 4 weeks
Combining records	1 h/w x 4 weeks
Tumor registry	1 h/w x 4 weeks
Correspondence	0.25 h/w x 4 weeks
Record completion	10.75 h/w x 4 weeks
Certificates	3.25 h/w x 4 weeks
Supervisory	5 h/w x 4 weeks
Transcription	0.10 h/record x 620 records
Coding	0.12 h/record x 850 records

Subtotal outpatient/ ambulatory surgery

Total hours worked

2. What percentage of the total hours is spent in each category of inpatient records, and what percentage is spent in inpatient, emergency department, general clinical, and outpatient/ambulatory surgery records? Round to two decimal places.

Service/Area	% of Time Worked
Pediatrics	
Obstetrics	
Psychiatric	
Newborn	
Medicine	
Surgery	
All inpatient records	
ED records	
General clinic records	
Outpatient/ambulatory surgery records	

Exercise 9.5

Your physician clinic's chief financial officer has determined that it costs the clinic $3.75 per telephone call for the receptionist to set up an appointment with a physician in the clinic compared to $1.50 per online request to set up an appointment. What would the cost savings be if, during one day at the clinic, 150 patient appointments were arranged by online request rather than by telephone?

Exercise 9.6

1. The Health Information Committee has requested information about the electronic signature system being used in your facility. They would like to know the locations where physicians are accessing the system. Review the information in the table below and determine the percentage of use from each site. Round to one decimal place.

Community Hospital
Electronic Signature System
250 physicians on staff; 231 using the system

Site	No. of Physicians Using the System at This Site	% of Physicians Using the System at This Site
Medicine, 2 West	45	
Medicine, 2 East	35	
Pediatrics, 3 West	20	
Obstetrics, 1 West	9	
Physician's lounge	65	
HIM department	42	
Physician home	15	

2. What is the percentage of physicians not using the electronic signature system? Round to one decimal place.

Exercise 9.7

Loose sheets continue to come to the HIM department even after the implementation of a hybrid electronic health record. Using the data provided in the table, compute the data requested below.

Community Hospital
Health Information Services
Loose Sheet Report
July 20XX

Department	Week #1	Week #2	Week #3	Week #4	Total	Proportion
Lab	27	34	48	54		
Radiology	15	21	26	42		
Pathology	25	26	28	31		
Nursing	17	22	36	41		
Physical therapy	5	4	2	12		
Miscellaneous	20	21	22	26		
Totals						

1. The totals for each department and each week:

2. The proportion of loose sheets received from each department:

Productivity

Productivity is defined as a unit of performance defined by management in quantitative standards. Productivity allows organizations to measure how well the organization converts input into output, or labor into a product or service.

Most HIM departments have productivity standards for different areas in the department. For example, in the coding section, a productivity standard may be that employees should code four inpatient records per hour. In a 7.5 hour workday (taking into account breaks the employee will take), 30 inpatient records would be coded per day. But how does the HIM manager or supervisor know how many records should be coded in a day? A number of factors influence this decision. Some things the supervisor should consider are:

- Does the coder do anything in addition to coding, such as abstracting, answering the phone, or obtaining additional information about the diagnoses and procedures?

- What kinds of records is the coder coding? Are they long lengths of stay or short? Are they complex cases or relatively simple cases to code?

In their article in the *Journal of AHIMA*, P. J. Miller and F. Waterstraat suggested two simple formulas that accurately calculate labor productivity (Miller and Waterstraat 2004):

$$Completed\ work = Total\ work\ output - Defective\ work$$

and

$$Labor\ productivity = \frac{Completed\ work}{Hours\ worked\ to\ produce\ total\ work\ output}$$

Determining the total work output and the hours worked is clear; however, determining the defective work involves auditing the work to determine if any work is defective. Miller and Waterstraat describe three ways to audit employees' work output. First, the manager could perform a review of all the work performed; second, the manager could perform a review of work chosen through a random sample; or third, the manager could use a fixed-percent random sample audit. The last suggestion is the easiest. This method requires the manager to select a fixed percent of total work for each employee to review. The manager also has a predetermined quality standard in mind and then reviews the work and classifies it as completed work or defective work. Additional work could be reviewed if more information is needed to determine the type of defect or until all the work has been reviewed.

Table 9.2 shows the calculation for determining inpatient coding productivity for one month.

Notice in table 9.2 that Coder D's average work output is 4.69 records per hour ($\frac{work\ output}{total\ hours\ worked} = \frac{375}{80} = 4.69$). However, after auditing the work, it was determined that 240 of those records were coded accurately (completed work output). Coder D's completed work is really 3.00 ($\frac{240}{80} = 3.00$).

Staffing Levels

Healthcare organizations use a variety of methods to determine appropriate staffing levels. For example, many outpatient facilities use patient encounters per **full-time equivalent employee** (FTE) per month. A patient encounter is any personal contact between a patient and a physician or other person authorized to furnish healthcare services for the diagnosis or treatment of the patient. These may include laboratory services, x-ray services, physical therapy, and other ancillary services.

The staffing level is determined by dividing the number of patient encounters by the expected productivity. An FTE is the total number of workers, including part-time, in an area as the equivalent of full-time positions. The number of FTEs does not always equal the actual number of employees because two or more part-time employees might equal one FTE.

$$\frac{Patient\ encounters}{Productivity} = Number\ of\ FTEs\ needed$$

Example: A small physician clinic experiences 300 patient encounters per day. A coder is expected to code 100 records per day. To determine the number of coders needed, divide 300 by 100. Thus, three coders are needed to perform the coding for the physician clinic each day.

Table 9.2.   Inpatient Coding Productivity Calculation for One Month

Coder	Work Output (all records coded)	Total Hours Worked	Average Work Output per Hour	Completed Work Percentage	Completed Work Output (records coded accurately)	Completed Work per Hours Worked
A	500	140	3.57	91%	455	3.25
B	475	140	3.39	96%	456	3.26
C	300	80	3.75	80%	240	3.00
D	375	80	4.69	64%	240	3.00
Department Average	^		3.69			3.13

Work Output: number of work units as recorded by the employee or the process

Total Hours Worked: number of hours worked by the employee to produce work, which does not include time on meals, breaks, and meetings

Average Work Output per Hour: work output divided by total hours worked

Completed Work Percentage: percentage of completed work from audit

Completed Work Output: work output multiplied by completed work percentage

Completed Work per Hours Worked: completed work output divided by total hours worked

Hospital HIM departments often use discharges as their method to determine staff levels.

Example: To determine the number of employees needed in a coding section, the health information manager first multiplies the average number of inpatient records coded per hour (6) by the number of hours in the workday (7.5), which amounts to 45 records coded per day. Hospital discharges numbered approximately 55 inpatients per day. Based on this number, the manager then calculated that she needed 1.2 FTEs to accomplish the coding task.

$$\frac{55}{45} = 1.2 \text{ FTE}$$

In this example, the manager would need one full-time employee plus one .2 FTE, which is computed as 40 hours per week multiplied by .2. Thus, she would need another employee to work eight hours per week to handle the workload.

Handy Tip: When computing FTE, the manager does not ordinarily round up or down. The reason is that managers must justify the need for any employees. The administration would only want to approve a .2 person because a full-time employee is not needed to perform the work.

Exercise 9.8

Community Physician's Clinic is a large clinic with 85 physicians. They treat about 8,600 patients each week. Coders are expected to code 100 clinic records each day. How many FTEs are needed to code these records?

Exercise 9.9

1. Community Hospital wants to make the transition to an electronic data management system. The process will involve scanning 5,000 inpatient records, 2,000 outpatient records, and 1,500 ED records into the new system. The hospital estimates that there are 30 pages per inpatient record, four pages per outpatient record, and three pages per ED record. Assuming that one scanning clerk can scan 1,500 pages per day, how many days will it take to complete the transition?

2. The HIM Department would like to complete this project in 30 days. How many FTEs will the HIM Department manager need to hire to complete this in a month?

3. Use the information in the table below to answer the following questions. Each employee worked eight-hour days during the 21 workdays in September. Round all answers to two decimal places.

   a. What percentage of the total number of records did each employee code during the month?
   b. How many records is each coder coding each workday?
   c. How many records is each coder coding per hour? (Use an 8-hour workday.)
   d. How many minutes does it take each coder to code one record?
   e. What percentage of records is not passing the quality screens for each coder?

Community Hospital
Health Information Management Department
Coding Section—Productive and Quality Audit Reports
September 20XX

Coder	No. of Records Coded	No. of Records Not Passing Quality Screens
A	425	4
B	502	3
C	373	11

Exercise 9.9 (continued)

Answers:

a. What percentage of the total number of records did each employee code during the month?

Coder A:

Coder B:

Coder C:

b. How many records is each coder coding each workday?

Coder A:

Coder B:

Coder C:

c. How many records is each coder coding per hour?

Coder A:

Coder B:

Coder C:

d. How many minutes does it take each coder to code one record?

Coder A:

Coder B:

Coder C:

(continued on next page)

Exercise 9.9 (continued)

e. What percentage of records is not passing the quality screens for each coder?

Coder A:

Coder B:

Coder C:

Budgets

If you are responsible for supervising a group of employees, you will most likely also be responsible for budgeting. Usually health information departments are involved with expense and capital budgets.

A **budget** is a plan that converts the organization's goals and objectives into targets for revenue and spending. Planning for the budget begins several months before the facility's **fiscal year** begins. During the planning process, the HIM supervisor uses skills learned in statistics to help approximate the department's expenses for the coming year. Departmental expenses may include employee wages and benefits, supplies, travel and education, membership dues, subscriptions, postage, copying, and equipment maintenance contracts.

The HIM department may also generate some revenue for the department, for example, if it is responsible for the ROI activity or provides a transcription or coding service for the hospital's physicians.

> **Handy Tip:** A fiscal year is a consecutive twelve-month period used by an organization as its accounting period. The fiscal year does not have to be a calendar year. For example, the U.S. government's fiscal year begins October 1 and ends September 30. It can be any twelve-month period.

Operational Budget

During the year, usually each month, a department director receives budget reports showing amounts budgeted and actual amounts spent. This report generally alerts the department director as to whether or not he or she is over or under budget. Any differences between the budgeted amount and the amount actually spent are called variances. As will be discussed in chapter 10, a variance is a disagreement between two parts. The variance can be used as a device to monitor the department's activities. Budgets also may be available on the organization's Intranet for viewing at any time. This is an easy way for the manager to stay aware of his or her department's budget.

The department director should check the budget report at least each month to determine whether any adjustments must be made in order to stay within the budget. Often the director may be required to explain why the department is over or under budget. This assessment of a department's financial transactions to identify differences between the budget amount and the actual amount of a line item is called a variance analysis.

To determine the variance, subtract the budgeted amount from the actual amount and then divide the difference by the budgeted amount.

Item	Budget	Actual	Variance
Supplies	$3,000	$4,000	($1,000)
Education/training	$1,000	$2,000	($1,000)

Using the information in the preceding table, the variance for supplies is $1,000, or 33.3 percent, over budget.

$$\$4,000 - \$3,000 = \$1,000$$
$$\frac{(\$1,000 \times 100)}{\$3,000} = 33.3\%$$

The variance for education and training is $1,000, or 100 percent, over budget.

$$\$2,000 - \$1,000 = \$1,000$$
$$\frac{(\$1,000 \times 100)}{\$1,000} = 100\%$$

The variances computed above are examples of unfavorable variances, that is, the amounts spent were more than the amounts budgeted.

Favorable variances occur when the amounts actually spent are less than or equal to the amounts budgeted, as shown in the table below.

Item	Budget	Actual	Variance
Supplies	$10,000	$8,000	$2,000
Education/training	$3,500	$2,000	$1,500

In this example, the variance for supplies is $2,000, or 20 percent, under budget.

$$\$10,000 - \$8,000 = \$2,000$$
$$\frac{(\$2,000 \times 100)}{\$10,000} = 20\%$$

The variance for education and training is $1,500, or 42.9 percent, under budget

$$\$3,500 - \$2,000 = \$1,500$$
$$\frac{(\$1,500 \times 100)}{\$3,500} = 42.9\%$$

Capital Budget

The capital budget accounts for the major assets the facility will purchase during the fiscal year, for example, equipment for the HIM department. Capital budget items usually are "high-dollar" purchases. Each facility defines what "high-dollar" means. For example, one facility may consider any assets purchased at a cost of more than $500 to be part of the capital budget.

Moreover, items included in a capital budget usually have a "life" of more than one year; that is, each item's usefulness should last longer than a year. Occasionally, the health information technician (HIT) is involved in assisting the department director in a cost justification for the capital budget. This is very important because only a certain amount of dollars can be allocated to the facility's departments and supervisors wish to have their projects approved. The department director may ask the supervisor to calculate the **payback period** of the project. The payback period provides information on how long it will take the project to recover its costs. The formula is:

$$\frac{Total\ cost\ of\ project}{Annual\ incremental\ cash\ flow}$$

The annual incremental cash flow refers to the savings that a department realizes from the project. For example, if the HIM department needs a new copy machine, the department director may ask the department supervisor to determine, first, how much a new copy machine costs and, then, what kind of savings would be realized from the purchase of a new machine. The supervisor would investigate the cost from different vendors and then calculate an estimate of the savings. Savings considerations might include the time not spent recopying pages, fixing the copy machine, or releasing papers trapped in the machine, as well as the cost of additional paper.

> **Example:** A new copy machine costs $3,000, and the department will realize a savings of $1,000 per year. The payback period is calculated as $\frac{\$3,000}{\$1,000} = 3$ years. There are some disadvantages to using the payback period because it assumes that there will always be the same amount of savings each year. In this example, it is possible that the savings may be less in the second or third year of use due to the aging of the equipment.

Another useful way that department supervisors determine cost justification is by the **return on investment** (ROI). ROI provides information on the rate at which cash is recovered from an investment project. The formula for computing ROI is:

$$\frac{Average\ annual\ incremental\ cash\ flow}{Total\ cost\ of\ the\ project}$$

Using the figures in the example above, the calculation is:

$$\frac{\$1,000 \times 100}{\$3,000} = 33.3\%$$

If 33.3 percent is greater than the facility's required rate of return, the copy machine may be a good investment. Other, more complex formulae are used to determine whether a particular project or major item can be undertaken; however, these formulae are generally performed by the facility's financial department.

Exercise 9.10

Complete the following exercises.

1. In deciding whether to purchase or lease a new dictation system, the HIM supervisor calculates the payback period. The hospital's required payback period is three years. If the equipment costs $28,000 and generates $3,500 per year in savings, what would be the payback period for this equipment? Should the department purchase this equipment?

2. The coding section in the HIM department shows its first-quarter budget analysis as having an expected cost of operation of $62,000. However, the actual cost of operation was $76,000. Calculate the budget variance. Round to one decimal place.

Verification of Statistical Reports

Many statistical reports in healthcare settings are computer-generated. However, a computer can only calculate statistics from the data that are entered. Standardization of terminology, data elements, and formulas from sources such as those found in appendix A will produce data that are more reliable and useful.

When a computerized statistical report is received, the HIM professional should examine it carefully. For example, he or she should verify the total number of discharges listed in a report from coded records and compare it against the total number of discharges according to the census data. Do the totals match? If not, it is important to find out why. Perhaps one of the discharges was not coded. Moreover, computerized statistical reports often give only whole numbers. Thus, the HIM professional may need to calculate certain statistics (for example, death rates) and carry them out to the second decimal place to make the information more valuable to administration or medical staff. Tables or graphs can be created to display a portion of a computerized statistical report. (See chapter 11.)

Computerized Discharge Reports

Figure 9.1 on page 154 shows a sample computerized discharge analysis report indicating that the average length of stay (ALOS) of total patients is 7.25 days. To verify this information, use your knowledge of ALOS and recalculate. The calculation is:

$$\frac{4,713}{650} = 7.25$$

Figure 9.1.   Computerized Discharge Analysis Report

*** YOUR UTILIZATION PROGRAM ***

SERVICE	TOTAL			AGE ANALYSIS						PATIENTS OPERATED	EMERGENCY ADMISSIONS	CONSULTATION	
				0-13 YEARS		14-64 YEARS		65 AND OVER				NO. OF PATIENTS	NUMBER RECEIVED
	PATIENTS	DAYS	AVG. STAY	PAT.	DAYS	PAT.	DAYS	PAT.	DAYS				
1	2	3	4	5	6	7	8	9	10	11	12	13	14
MEDICINE	204	1880	9.2	1	2	161	1300	42	578	170	3	128	209
CARDIOLOGY	60	626	10.4			43	436	17	190	44	1	17	21
ENDOCRINOLOGY	2	23	11.5			2	23			2		2	3
GASTROENTEROL	13	99	7.6			13	99			13		6	11
ONCOLOGY	17	178	10.5			10	112	7	66	16		8	15
PULMONARY MED	4	40	10.0			4	40			4		1	1
PSYCHIATRY	3	17	5.7			2	14	1	3	1		2	6
OB-LIVE BIR	26	114	4.4			26	114			25		2	3
OB-NOT DELIV	9	23	2.6			9	23			4			
OB-ABOR FETUS	15	26	1.7			15	26			15		1	1
GYNECOLOGY	33	125	3.8			33	125			31		5	11
NEWBORN	25	130	5.2	25	130					6			
PED MED	47	265	5.6	44	217	3	48			30	1	8	11
PED SURG	5	11	2.2	4	9	1	2			5		2	2
PED ORTHO	5	27	5.4	2	10	3	17			5		4	5
PED RHINOLARYN	2	3	1.5	1	1	1	2			1		1	1
PED OPHTH	1	2	2.0	1	2					1		1	1
PED UROL	1	1	1.0	1	1					1			
SURGERY	35	222	6.3	1	2	31	190	3	30	34	2	13	18
CV SURG	7	74	10.6			6	72	1	2	7		4	5
ORTHOPEDICS	77	551	7.2	1	11	73	506	3	34	74	1	51	78
PLAS SURG	4	8	2.0			4	8			4		1	1
PROCTOLOGY	1	5	5.0			1	5			1			
ORAL SURG-ADU	3	6	2.0			3	6			3			
UROLOGY	23	172	7.5			18	131	5	41	22		12	16
OPHTHALMOLOGY	5	18	3.6			3	9	2	9	5		2	2
RHINOLARYNG	5	17	3.4	1	1	3	13	1	3	5		1	1
ADULT T & A	2	4	2.0			2	4			2			
PED T & A	1	1	1.0	1	1					1			
PODIATRY	15	45	3.0			14	41	1	4	15		5	6
TOTALS INC / NB	650	4713	7.3	83	387	484	3366	83	960	547	8	277	428
LESS NEWBORNS	25	130											
TOTALS EXC / NB	625	4583											

| TOTAL CASES | AVG. STAY | TRANSFERRED TO | | | | | LENGTH OF STAY DISTRIBUTION | | | |
| | | OTHER HOSP. | SNF | | HOME CARE | | 1 – 3 DAYS | 4 – 14 DAYS | 15 – 30 DAYS | OVER 30 DAYS |
			UNDER 64	65 AND OVER	UNDER 64	65 AND OVER				
625	7.3	8	1	7			28%	62%	10%	%

| % OF PATIENTS OPERATED | % OF EMERG ADM. | % OF PATIENTS W/ CONS | AVG. # OF CONS | TRANSFER RATE | | |
				TO OTHER HOSP.	TO SNF	TO HOME CARE
84%	01%	43%	2	1.2%	1.2%	

Figure 9.1. Computerized Discharge Analysis Report *(continued)*

HOSP # XXXX   JAN 20XX   PAGE 1

	DISCHARGE STATUS							PAYMENT STATUS							
			DEATHS					COMMERCIAL		BLUE CROSS		MEDICAID		MEDICARE	
ALIVE STATUS	A M A	TRANSFER	EXP NO AUT	EXP AUT	COR. CASE NO AUT	AUT	PAT.	DAYS	PAT.	DAYS	PAT.	DAYS	PAT.	DAYS	
15	16	17	18	19	20	21	22	23	24	25	26	27	28	29
184	4	14	2				39	323	72	625	28	172	53	700
56		2	1	1			9	60	20	235	5	43	24	273
2											1	9	1	14
13							3	20	7	54	1	11	2	14
14			3				4	38	4	44	2	30	7	66
4							3	33			1	7		
		3					1	5	1	9			1	3
26							2	14	7	34	2	52		
9							1	1	1	1	6	20		
15							2	4	9	14	2	5		
33							7	22	16	51	10	52		
25							2	11	6	33	13	55		
47							12	73	16	91	18	100		
5							2	3	3	8				
5							3	19	1	7				
2									2	3				
1									1	2				
1											1	1		
33			1		1		11	57	19	107			4	38
6		1					2	22	2	21			3	31
76		1					29	233	20	161	8	21	4	46
4									3	7	1	1		
1							1	5						
3									3	6				
23							5	27	10	73	2	19	5	41
5									3	9			2	9
5							2	3	2	11			1	3
2									2	4				
1							1	1						
15							4	11	7	23	3	7	1	4
616		21			2			985		1633		605		1242
	4		7				145		237		114		108	

DEATHS							OTHER PAYMENT STATUS							
GROSS DEATH RATE	NET DEATH RATE	GROSS AUT. RATE	NET AUT. RATE	COR CASES	POST-OP		SELF-PAY		WORK-COMP		FREE OTHER – GOV		UMW	
							PAT	DAYS	PAT	DAYS	PAT	DAYS	PAT	DAYS
01%	01%	22%	22%				26	124	18	107	1	9		

DAY OF WEEK OF ADMISSION							DAY OF WEEK OF DISCHARGE						
SUN	MON	TUES	WED	THURS	FRI	SAT	SUN	MON	TUES	WED	THURS	FRI	SAT
13%	13%	18%	15%	17%	14%	10%	07%	12%	14%	19%	14%	19%	15%

Another verification can be done by adding the percentages given for the day-of-the-week admissions and the day-of-the-week discharges to make certain they add up to 100 percent. In the computerized statistical report in figure 9.1, they do add up to 100 percent (13 + 13 + 18 + 15 + 17 + 14 + 10 = l00, and 7 + 12 + 14 + 19 + 14 + 19 + 15 = 100). These data could be presented in the form of a **pie chart**. (See chapter 11.)

Reports such as the one shown in figure 9.1 are useful to hospital administrators; this type of review can give some insights into the resources and services used in the facility.

Example: The psychiatrists on staff are requesting that a new 15-bed psychiatry wing be built to accommodate their patients. The administrator could look at this report and see that there were only three psychiatry patients in this month. If this is normal for the hospital, then can the administration justify this expense? Most likely not. However, some other questions that could be posed by administration are: Would adding a separate psychiatry wing increase the number of admissions to the hospital? How many psychiatrists are in the community and would they admit their patients to our hospital if there were more beds? Is there something else happening in the community that could increase the number of psychiatry admissions?

Example: If the orthopedists asked for a new treatment room, the administrator can see that 77 patients were seen in this month. Certainly, additional comparison reports would need to be done to ascertain the number of patients seen by the orthopedists before a decision is made. However, these types of reports can serve as a baseline to begin collecting other types of data for decision-making projects.

Computerized Financial Statistical Reports

Computers are also used to compile various financial statistical reports. A sample computerized financial report is shown in figure 9.2.

Computerized Readmission Rate Reports

Figure 9.3 shows an example of a computerized readmission rate report. This type of report delineates inpatients by medical service and calculates each medical service's readmission rate.

Case-Mix Index Report

Figure 9.4 shows a sample of a computerized case-mix index report. This report portrays the facility's case-mix index for all financial classes for the month and the fiscal year to date. It also shows the case-mix index for Medicare-only patients. The case-mix index refers to the average relative weight of all cases treated at a given facility or by a given physician, which reflects the resource intensity or clinical severity of a specific group in relation to the other groups in the classification system. Case-mix is always reported with four decimal points. The formula for computing case-mix is:

$$\frac{\textit{Sum of the weights of MS-DRGs (Medicare severity diagnosis-related groups) for patients discharged during a given period}}{\textit{Total number of patients discharged}}$$

Figure 9.2.   Computerized Financial Report

	Community Hospital Most Frequent MS-DRGs by Financial Class Medicare Patients Only Annual Report 20XX				
MS-DRG	**MS-DRG Title**	**No. of Pts**	**Pt. Days**	**ALOS**	**Tot. Charges**
293	Heart failure & shock w/o CC/MCC	216	1,252	5.8	$2,125,018.00
066	Intracranial hemorrhage or cerebral infarction w/o CC/MCC	141	1,009	7.2	$1,798,011.89
470	Major joint replacement or reattachment of lower extremity w/o MCC	136	926	6.8	$2,601,090.62
195	Simple pneumonia & pleurisy w/o CC/MCC	117	807	6.9	$1,271,445.45
192	Chronic obstructive pulmonary disease w/o CC/MCC	98	579	5.9	$920,071.41
378	G.I. hemorrhage w CC	94	487	5.2	$964,597.03
178	Respiratory infections & inflammations w CC	88	905	10.3	$1,656,856.52
330	Major small & large bowel procedures w CC	88	1,092	12.4	$2,493,260.52
391	Esophagitis, gastroent & misc digest disorders w MCC	86	324	3.8	$560,025.93
469	Major joint replacement or reattachment of lower extremity w MCC	81	617	7.6	$1,329,055.73
309	Cardiac arrhythmia & conduction disorders w CC	71	290	4.1	$506,803.44
311	Angina pectoris	70	234	3.3	$466,286.80
872	Septicemia w/o MV 96+ hours w/o MCC	69	619	9.0	$1,209,069.85
640	Nutritional & misc metabolic disorders w MCC	63	366	5.8	$532,230.77
286	Circulatory disorders except AMI, w card cath w MCC	56	248	4.4	$687,146.08
068	Nonspecific cva & precerebral occlusion w/o infarct w/o MCC	52	158	3.0	$336,667.38
280	Acute myocardial infarction, discharged alive w MCC	51	328	6.4	$790,417.76
689	Kidney & urinary tract infections w MCC	47	240	5.1	$367,789.93
189	Pulmonary edema & respiratory failure	43	369	8.6	$707,485.01
839	Chemo w acute leukemia as sdx w/o CC/MCC	41	85	2.1	$198,692.68
389	G.I. obstruction w CC	39	235	6.0	$386,509.40
244	Permanent cardiac pacemaker implant w/o CC/MCC	33	146	4.4	$592,506.88
394	Other digestive system diagnoses w CC	33	218	6.6	$427,499.12
315	Other circulatory system diagnoses w CC	31	189	6.1	$447,102.64

(continued on next page)

Figure 9.2.   Computerized Financial Report *(continued)*

Community Hospital **Most Frequent MS-DRGs by Financial Class** **Medicare Patients Only** **Annual Report 20XX**					
MS-DRG	**MS-DRG Title**	**No. of Pts**	**Pt. Days**	**ALOS**	**Tot. Charges**
208	Respiratory system diagnosis w ventilator support <96 hours	31	387	12.5	$1,215,601.28
842	Lymphoma & non-acute leukemia w/o CC/MCC	1	4	4.0	$4,011.41
844	Other myeloprolif dis or poorly diff neopl diag w CC	1	23	23.0	$45,480.70
876	O.R. procedure w principal diagnoses of mental illness	1	20	20.0	$26,289.88
883	Disorders of personality & impulse control	1	19	19.0	$15,508.06
958	Other O.R. procedures for multiple significant trauma w CC	1	14	14.0	$35,775.10
913	Traumatic injury w MCC	1	4	4.0	$5,560.30
916	Allergic reactions w/o MCC	1	5	5.0	$10,687.30
922	Other injury, poisoning & toxic effect diag w MCC	1	2	2.0	$6,522.35
923	Other injury, poisoning & toxic effect diag w/o MCC	1	2	2.0	$3,161.58
941	O.R. proc w diagnoses of other contact w health services w/o CC/MCC	1	3	3.0	$3,302.98
947	Signs & symptoms w MCC	1	6	6.0	$9,279.07
264	Other circulatory system O.R. procedures	1	2	2.0	$23,031.87
956	Limb reattachment, hip & femur proc for multiple significant trauma	1	7	7.0	$21,149.70
959	Other O.R. procedures for multiple significant trauma w/o CC/MCC	1	5	5.0	$14,882.29
977	HIV w or w/o other related condition	1	4	4.0	$7,104.30
837	Other digestive system diagnoses w CC	1	10	10.0	$28,618.33
		1,891	12,240	6.5	$24,851,607.34

Figure 9.3.   Computerized Readmission Rate Report

Community Hospital Readmission Rate For Month End 10/20XX			
Case Type	**Number of Readmits**	**Number of Cases**	**Readmit Rate (%)**
I	188	2,046	9.18

Readmission Rate by Service For Month End 10/20XX				
Case Type	**Medical Service**	**Number of Readmits**	**Number of Cases**	**Readmit Rate (%)**
I	ABS		3	.00
I	ABT		1	.00
I	ALL		1	.00
I	CRD	10	277	3.61
I	CVS	10	84	11.90
I	DLC	5	70	7.14
I	DLN		16	.00
I	DLR		53	.00
I	END		2	.00
I	FPR	5	75	6.66
I	GI	5	27	18.51
I	GYN	1	68	1.47
I	INF	1	8	12.50
I	MED	59	511	11.54
I	MON	26	67	38.80
I	NB	1	129	.77
I	NEU	1	4	25.00
I	NIC		21	.00
I	NIN		1	.00
I	NPH	42	162	25.92
I	NRS		25	.00
I	OB	3	80	3.75
I	ONR		1	.00
I	OPH		1	.00
I	ORS	2	14	14.28
I	ORT	4	84	4.76

(continued on next page)

Figure 9.3.   Computerized Readmission Rate Report *(continued)*

Case Type	Medical Service	Number of Readmits	Number of Cases	Readmit Rate
I	OTO		11	.00
I	PED	1	55	1.81
I	PPA	1	2	50.00
I	PUL		4	.00
I	RON	2	2	100.00
I	RPL		11	.00
I	SUR	4	71	5.63
I	THS	3	37	8.10
I	URO	1	42	2.38
I	VSS	1	26	3.84
I			2,046	

Figure 9.4.   Computerized Case-Mix Index Report

Community Hospital Case-Mix Index Report—All Financial Classes For Fiscal Year to Date, 20XX		
Total Weight	**Number of Cases**	**Case-Mix Index**
6831.0912	3,230	2.1148
Case Mix Index Report—Medicare Only For Fiscal Year to Date, 20XX		
Total Weight	**Number of Cases**	**Case-Mix Index**
2915.2882	1,367	2.1326
Case Mix Index Report—All Financial Classes For Month End 10/20XX		
Total Weight	**Number of Cases**	**Case-Mix Index**
3396.8017	1,626	2.0890
Case Mix Index Report—Medicare Only For Month End 10/20XX		
Total Weight	**Number of Cases**	**Case-Mix Index**
1364.1506	658	2.0731

Physician Reports

Healthcare organizations have always been interested in finding effective ways of measuring the utilization of services provided by physicians. One approach commonly used to analyze services is profiling. **Profiling** is defined as a measurement of the quality, utilization, and cost of medical resources provided by physicians that is made by employers, third-party payers, government entities, and other purchasers of healthcare. Figure 9.5 is a report of a facility's physician profile. This report lists important information about how physicians use the services of the facility. This is important to the organization's administration because they need to know if physician services are increasing or decreasing. If services are increasing, the question of additional equipment or staff needs to be addressed; if they are decreasing, the question of why becomes paramount.

Exercise 9.11

Complete the following exercises using the reports in figures 9.1 through 9.4

1. The report in figure 9.1 gives the gross death rate (hospital death rate) as .01 percent. Recalculate this rate and round to the second decimal place.

2. Recalculate the gross autopsy rate in figure 9.1. Round your answer to the second decimal place.

3. In figure 9.2 which Medicare severity diagnosis-related group (MS-DRG) has the greatest ALOS?

4. Recalculate the readmission rates for the medical services and the overall rate in figure 9.3 to verify their accuracy. Which readmission rates were not accurate? Round your answers to two decimal points.

5. Recalculate the rates in figure 9.4 to verify their accuracy. Are there any that were calculated incorrectly? If so, which ones? How many Medicare patients were discharged during the fiscal year to date? What month end was this report calculated?

Spreadsheets

Numerous statistical software packages are available for the creation of spreadsheets. Spreadsheets, or worksheets, allow you to enter text, numbers, and formulas to assist in calculations.

A spreadsheet consists of columns lettered across the top of the document and rows numbered down the left side of the document. The intersections of columns and rows form cells, which are the basic units for storing data.

Each software package varies slightly in method. Most packages perform basic arithmetic functions as well as many of the statistical calculations discussed in this book. Various add-in features allow for data sorting, formatting for printing data, and even graphical

Figure 9.5.   Physician Profile

Atten. Phys.	Total						Deaths						Pts. Receiving Consults			
	Cases	Surg Cases	Days	ESD Pts.	ALOS	Preop LOS	TOT	% of Dths	Post Op	W/in 48 hrs	Aut Cas	Cor Cas	Tot Pts	Cons Rec'd	Avg Cons	Cons Rate
01000	202	18	1111	69	5.5	3.1	12	5.9	1		1		72	104	1.4	36%
01005	182	21	1911	49	105	5.5	14	7.7		2	1		93	146	1.6	51%
01006	259	42	2719	88	10.3	4.5	15	5.8	2	2	1		122	175	1.4	47%
01009	242	29	2250	79	9.3	3.8	18	7.4	1	3	1	1	117	162	1.4	48%
04000	53	6	509	9	9.6	4.0	4	7.5		1	1		30	43	1.4	57%
10125	1	1	2		2.0	1.0										
15000	3	3	31	1	10.3	1.0							1	1	1.0	33%
15002	76	10	737	19	9.7	4.6	4	5.3		1	1		55	93	1.7	72%
15006	188	18	1354	64	7.2	5.6	7	3.7	1	1	1	1	77	103	1.3	41%
15007	2		18	2	9.0											
15008	95	5	751	32	7.9	4.0	4	4.2			2		55	76	1.4	58%
Total	**1,303**	**153**	**11,393**	**412**	**8.7**	**3.7**	**78**	**6.0**	**5**	**10**	**8**	**2**	**622**	**903**	**1.4**	**48%**

interface. Most software packages contain a help section and a tutorial to assist the novice. The best way to gain proficiency with any software package is to "just do it" and practice, practice, practice.

Exercise 9.12

Complete the following spreadsheets.

1. Using Worksheet No. 1 in exercise 3.9 on page 36, create a computerized spreadsheet to calculate the patient census.

2. Using the table in exercise 5.4 on page 61, which lists 15 patients by name, age, clinical service, and LOS, create a computerized spreadsheet to calculate the ALOS.

Chapter 9 Test

Complete the following exercises.

1. If your HIM department has 100,000 active medical records and you received 5,352 requests for records within a six-month period, what is the request rate for the past six months? Round to two decimal points.

2. Of the 5,352 requests for medical records in the question above, 4,257 were located within the 20-minute time frame established by the supervisor as a quality improvement indicator. What is the rate of compliance in answering requests for records? Round to two decimal points.

3. Community Health Center, a new patient clinic in your town serving only underinsured and uninsured patients, has asked you to help its HIM department get started. Calculate the number of new shelving units needed for a medical record filing system based on 8 shelves per unit at 36 inches per shelf. The average record size equals .30 inches, and the center anticipates seeing 4,500 patients the first year.

4. After one month of operation, the health information services at Community Health Center determined that there were two records misfiled out of the 450 active records. What is the filing accuracy rate for this area? Round to one decimal point.

5. An employee currently earning $10.85 per hour has been awarded a 3.5 percent merit raise. What will the employee's hourly salary be with this increase?

6. It takes approximately 15 minutes to code one record. How many personnel hours would be needed to code 1,424 discharges for the month?

(continued on next page)

Chapter 9 Test (continued)

7. A coding supervisor must determine the number of full-time equivalents (FTEs) needed to code 500 discharges per week. If it takes an average of 20 minutes to code each record and each coder works 7.5 productive hours per day, how many FTEs will the coding supervisor need?

8. The HIM Department at Community Hospital will experience a 15 percent increase in the number of discharges coded per day as the result of opening a cardiac clinic in the facility. The 15 percent increase is projected to be 100 additional records per day. The standard time to code this type of record is 10 minutes. Compute the number of FTEs required to handle this increased volume in coding based on a seven-hour productive day.

9. The HIM coding supervisor over the coding section agrees to pay a new graduate $11.00 per hour. This is a full-time coding position at 2,080 hours per year. The cost for a full-time employee's fringe benefits is 24 percent of the employee's salary. How much must the supervisor budget for the employee's salary and fringe benefits?

10. The same supervisor in #9 agreed to increase the salary of the employee to $13.00 per hour once she passed her RHIT exam. Three months after beginning her employment, the employee passed her RHIT exam. What will the new budget be for salary and fringe benefits?

11. The forms used in your coding area cost $100.00 per 1,000 forms for the first 2,000 and $50 for every 1,000 thereafter. If you need to order 5,000 forms, what is the total cost?

12. You currently lease scanning equipment at a cost of $1,500 per quarter and two copy machines at $120 each per month. What will you need to budget annually for this leased equipment?

13. What is the percent of variance for each item listed in the HIM department budget shown in the table below? Round to two decimal points.

Community Hospital
Health Information Department
Fiscal Year 20XX

Item	Budget Amount	Actual Amount	Variance/% of Variance
Supplies	$1,600	$1,595	
Outside temp service	$6,800	$7,200	
Travel	$1,500	$1,526	
Conference fees	$500	$455	
Postage	$1,000	$1,017	
Subscriptions	$325	$330	
Maintenance contracts	$1,500	$1,500	

Chapter 9 Test (continued)

14. All the patients who present to the emergency services department with a suspected acute myocardial infarction (AMI) are expected to receive an EKG within 10 minutes of their arrival. Of the 56 patients who had a suspected AMI during the last quarter, 32 had an EKG within the specified time frame. What was the rate of compliance? Round to two decimal places.

15. Last month, the release of information specialist received 232 requests for information. He was able to answer 176 within the specified time frame of five working days. What is the rate of compliance in answering requests within the specified time frame? Round to two decimal places.

16. Estimate the hospital charges for the patients listed in the table below based on an average cost of $950 per day.

Community Hospital

Patient Number	LOS	Estimated Charges
171819	3	
124785	4	
452362	5	
326578	8	
528615	9	
213624	12	
242628	10	
659832	5	
428231	3	
269761	5	

17. Last year, Community Hospital had 23,652 admissions. Of these 1,569 were readmissions. What is the hospital's readmission rate? Round to two decimal places.

18. In September, the hospital had three coders who coded 1,200 inpatient records, and 18 of the records failed the quality screens.
    a. What is the average number of records coded by each coder?
    b. What was the average number of records coded each working day (Monday through Friday at 21 workdays) in September? Round to two decimal points.
    c. What percentage of records passed the quality screens? Round to two decimal points.

(continued on next page)

Chapter 9 Test (continued)

19. At Community Hospital each full-time employee is required to work 2,080 hours annually. The table below shows the amount of time that five employees were absent from work over the past year. Use this information to answer the following questions. Round all answers to two decimal places.

    a. What is the total absentee rate for each employee?
    b. What is the sick leave rate for each employee?
    c. What is the total sick leave rate for this group of employees for the year?

Community Hospital
Health Information Management Department
Coding Section
Absentee Report
Annual Statistics 20XX

Employee Name	Vacation Hours Used	Sick Leave Hours Used
A	40	0
B	20	16
C	32	8
D	80	32
E	16	40

20. The coding department of a large physician clinic is interested in purchasing a software program that will edit claims before they are sent to the Billing Office. The license fee for the software is $52,000 per year. The software is expected to reduce the number of errors on claims and thus reduce the number of claims returned to the clinic for recoding. Currently, the department codes 32,600 physician visits per month and 450 claims are returned each month for recoding. The facility pays two FTEs in the Billing Office $11.50 per hour each to refile the returned claims. The software company promises that its software will reduce the number of returned claims by 90 percent.

    a. What is the rate of claims that are currently being returned for recoding each month? Round to two decimal places.
    b. How many claims would be returned after the installation of the software?
    c. If the clinic eliminated the two FTEs that handle the returned claims, what savings would it realize after installation of the software?
    d. What is the payback period?
    e. What is the return on investment?

Chapter 9 Test (continued)

21. What is physician profiling, and why is important to healthcare organizations?

22. Spreadsheet software programs allow you to enter text, numbers, and formulas to assist in calculations. True or false?

23. What is a hospital's case-mix index?

24. Using the information in the table below, calculate the case-mix index for each month in the first quarter at Community Hospital.

Community Hospital
First Quarter Statistics
Case-Mix-Report

	January	February	March
Total Discharges	2,012	1,983	2,112
Total weight	7156.2315	7733.7523	9715.2354
Case-mix Index			

Chapter 10
Descriptive Statistics in Healthcare

Objectives

At the conclusion of this chapter, you should be able to:

- Define descriptive statistics
- Define the terms rank, quartile, decile, and percentile
- Explain how and why percentiles are used
- Compute the percentile from an ungrouped distribution
- Define and compute the mean, median, and mode
- Define and differentiate among range, variance, and standard deviation
- Calculate range, variance, and standard deviation
- Define and compute correlation

Descriptive Statistics

Descriptive statistics are used to explain data in ways that are manageable and easily understood. The following sections discuss the basic concepts of rank, quartile, decile, percentile, measures of central tendency (mean, median, mode), measures of variation (range, variance, standard deviation), and correlation.

Frequency Distribution

Before studying measures in descriptive statistics, it would be useful to briefly cover two concepts: **variable and frequency distribution.** A variable is a characteristic that can have different values. For example, a person may be HIV negative or positive. The characteristic is HIV status and the values are negative and positive. Third-party payers, race, LOS, and services are examples of variables. Within each variable, there is more than one possible value. For example, third-party payers include numerous insurance companies. The variable is "third-party payer" while the values are the names of the organizations paying for services.

Because it is difficult to look at data in raw form, they are often summarized into frequency distributions. A frequency distribution shows the values that a variable can take and the number of observations associated with each value. Using the previous example, a facility conducting HIV testing may be interested in the number or frequency of HIV negative and positive individuals using their services. This information is valuable when seeking funding.

> **Example:** Table 10.1 below provides an example of a frequency distribution in which types of third-party payers are identified, along with the number of patients in an organization associated with each payer.

Rank

Rank denotes a score's position in a group relative to other scores organized in order of magnitude. For example, a rank of 50 means that a score is 50th from the beginning (or

Table 10.1.   Example of a Frequency Distribution by Number of Patients Discharged from Community Hospital by Third-Party Payer, June 20XX

Third-Party Payer	No. of Patients
Medicare	98
Medicaid	56
Tri-Care	23
Blue Cross	85
Mutual of Omaha	67
Other Private Payer	76
Total	405

end) of a series. The number of scores in a sequence is important in determining the significance of a rank. If there are only 60 scores, a rank of 50th is interpreted much differently than if there are 1,000 scores. For this reason, it may be more useful to express data as percentiles.

In ranked data, the position of the observation is more important than the number associated with it. For example, it is possible to list the major causes of death in the United States, along with the number of lives that each cause claimed. If the causes were ordered starting with the one that resulted in the greatest number of deaths and ending with the one that caused the fewest, and these were assigned consecutive integers, the data are said to be ranked.

Table 10.2 shows a report listing the fifteen leading causes of death in the United States in 2006. Note that cerebrovascular disease would be ranked third regardless of whether it causes 560,101 or 137,266 deaths.

Quartile

In addition to determining the rank of the score in a group, it can be helpful to divide data into smaller parts to better understand the relationship among scores. Data organized in order of magnitude can be divided into four equal parts, or quartiles. The first quartile includes the first 25% of the data, the second quartile extends to the median or one half of the data. The third quartile extends to 75% of the data.

Table 10.2. Fifteen Leading Causes of Death in the United States in 2006

Rank	Causes of Death	Total Deaths
1	Diseases of heart	629,191
2	Malignant neoplasms	560,102
3	Cerebrovascular diseases	137,265
4	Chronic lower respiratory diseases	124,614
5	Accidents (unintentional injuries)	117,748
6	Alzheimer's disease	72,914
7	Diabetes mellitus	72,507
8	Influenza and pneumonia	56,247
9	Nephritis, nephritic syndrome, and nephrosis	77,791
10	Septicemia	34,031
11	Intentional self-harm (suicide)	32,185
12	Chronic liver disease and cirrhosis	27,299
13	Essential hypertension and hypertensive renal disease	23,985
14	Parkinson's disease	19,660
15	Assault (homicide)	18,029

Decile

In similar fashion, deciles represent data divided into ten equal parts. The first decile corresponds to the 10th percentile and includes the first 10% of the scores; the second decile corresponds to the 20th percentile and includes the second 10% of the data, and so on.

Percentile

As quartiles divide scores into four equal parts and deciles into ten, percentiles separate the scores into 100 equal parts. If a person scores at the 54th percentile, his score is greater than or equal to 54% of all the scores in the group. This is called a percentile rank.

How and Why Percentiles Are Used

Percentiles help people understand their score relative to all scores from a group. If a student is told that she received a score of 34 on a test and she did not know how many points were possible, the 34 has no significance. However, if she is told that the score was in the 95th percentile, this would give a better understanding of the score compared to her peers; that is, only 5% of the class received a higher score.

To find the score that falls within a given percentile in a group of data arranged in order of magnitude:

1. Multiply the desired percentile's percentage by the total number of scores in the given group of scores (N). For example, the 38th percentile's percentage would be 38%. Likewise, the 90th percentile's percentage would be 90%.

2. This number indicates which score in the group will represent the desired percentile.

Example: The following numbers represent lengths of newborns in inches.

12, 12, 12, 13, 13, 15, 15, 16, 17, 18, 19, 20, 21, 21, 22, 22, 23, 23, 24, 25

$$N = 20$$

To find the 60th percentile:

1. Multiply 60% by 20 (N) = 12

2. Count up to the 12th score

3. The 60th percentile is 20

This means that 40% of the newborns were over 20 inches in length at birth.

On the other hand, if you want to know in what percentile a score is, take that score and divide the number of scores that are equal to and less than your score by the total number of scores and then multiply by 100.

Example: For instance, in the example above, suppose you want to find the percentile of the newborns that are over 17 inches in length. Take 9 (17 is the ninth score) divided by 20 (the N) × 100.

$$\left(\frac{9}{20}\right) \times 100 = 45^{\text{th}} \text{ percentile.}$$

17 falls in the 45th percentile. This means that 45% of the newborns are 17 inches or less in length at birth and 55% (100% − 45%) were over 17 inches in length at birth.

Exercise 10.1

1. Your instructor told you that you are in the 54th percentile in your class. This means that your score is greater than or equal to 54% of all the scores in the class. True or False?

2. Use the information below to find your percentile. Your score is 86.

Test scores out of 100 points

95	97
99	74
84	91
65	94
54	89
35	88
86	56
77	96
76	27
100	75
92	93

Measures of Central Tendency

In summarizing data, it is often useful to have a single *typical* number that is representative of the entire collection of data or specific population. Such numbers are customarily referred to as **measures of central tendency**. A common measure of central tendency is average or mean. It is sum of a set of numbers divided by the number of data points in the set of numbers. One of the most common examples of a mean or average in a healthcare facility involves **length of stay**, or LOS (number of days from admission to discharge that a patient stays in the hospital). The **average length of stay** (ALOS) was discussed in detail in chapter 5 and is discussed briefly in this chapter.

Three measures of central tendency are frequently used: mean, median, and mode. Each measure has advantages and disadvantages in describing a typical value.

Mean

The **mean** is the arithmetic average. It is common to use the term average to designate mean. It is computed by dividing the sum of all the scores (Σ) by the total number of scores (N).

Example: Seven hospital inpatients have the following lengths of stay: 2, 3, 4, 3, 5, 1, and 3 days. To construct a frequency distribution, all the values that the LOS can take are listed in ascending order (in this example, 1, 2, 3, 3, 3, 4, and 5) and the number of times a discharged patient had each LOS is entered. Table 10.3 shows the frequency distribution for this example. As the table shows, three patients were discharged with an LOS of three days each and the remaining four patients were discharged with an LOS of one, two, four, and five days each.

Table 10.3.   Frequency Distribution of Seven Hospital Inpatients

LOS	No. of Patients Discharged
1	1
2	1
3	3
4	1
5	1

Example: To obtain the mean, divide the total number of inpatient days ($1 + 2 + 3 + 3 + 3 + 4 + 5 = 21$) by the number of values (or frequency distribution), in this case, 7 inpatients. This gives a mean of three days. This may also be written as mean ($\bar{X}$) = 3 days.

The symbol $\bar{X}$ (pronounced "ex bar") is used to represent the mean in this formula

$$\frac{Total\ sum\ of\ all\ the\ values}{Number\ of\ the\ values\ involved} = \bar{X}$$

or

$$\frac{\Sigma\ scores}{N} = \frac{Sum\ of\ all\ scores}{Total\ number\ of\ scores}$$

Handy Tip: You may hear individuals refer to the average or mean as "The average age is 10 to 20." This is the wrong use of this statistic. In this example, they are referring to a range of ages, which may be the desired expression in some instances. However, the average is only one value.

The mean is the most common measure of central tendency. One of the advantages is that it is easy to compute. It is used as the basis for a large proportion of statistical tests. One disadvantage of the mean is that it is sensitive to extreme values, called **outliers** that may distort its representation of the typical value of a set of numbers. For example, if each of six women in a group weighed 110, 115, 120, 122, 125, and 227 pounds, the mean weight of the group would be $\frac{819}{6}$, or 136.5 pounds. However, given that five of the women weigh 125 pounds or less, the mean of this sample is not a very good indication of a typical observation. Thus, the more asymmetric or unequal the distribution, the less desirable it is to summarize the observations by using the mean.

Median

The **median** is the midpoint (center) of the distribution of values, or the point above and below which 50 percent of the values fall. The median value is obtained by arranging the numerical observations in ascending or descending order and then determining the middle value. This may be the middle observation (if there is an odd number of values) or a point halfway between the two middle values (if there is an even number of values).

To arrive at the median in an even-numbered distribution, add the two middle values together and divide by 2. When the two middle values are the same, the median is that value.

Example: The numbers in the LOS example used earlier are sequenced as follows:

1

2

3

3 ← median (midpoint)

3

4

5

The median is 3.

Example: The median weight of the women who weighed 110, 115, 120, 122, 125, and 227 pounds is shown as follows:

110

115

120

← median $\left(120 + 122 = \dfrac{242}{2} = 121 \right)$

122

125

227

The median is 121.

Handy Tip: The advantage to using the median as a measure of central tendency is that it is unaffected by outliers. The value of 121 pounds is much more representative of the fact that five out of the six women weigh 125 pounds or less than the mean value of 136.5 as seen in the example above.

The median is also often used in calculating length of stay in long-term care cases. As discussed in chapter 5, a long-stay patient's discharge days are allocated to the period in which he or she is discharged. Sometimes this can give a distorted average, especially on a monthly (rather than annual) basis.

Example: In March, a long-term care facility discharged 130 patients with a total length of stay of 1,267 days. The LOS for one of the patients was 365 days. The ALOS for all 130 patients was 9.8 days ($\frac{1,267}{130}$ = 9.75). If the stay of the one patient is removed from the total length of stay, the ALOS becomes 6.99 or 7.0 days (1,267 − 365 = $\frac{902}{129}$ = 6.99). Should one patient or a few patients in a population affect the average to this degree? Is the statistical computation meaningful for decision-making purposes? In this situation, the facility has two options:

- First, a notation can be made on the report that either the ALOS of 9.8 includes one patient who stayed 365 days or the ALOS of 7.0 excludes one patient who stayed 365 days. Both calculations can be made. Appropriate notes should be attached to the report to indicate the difference.

- Second, the computation using the median rather than the mean can be used. The individual lengths of stay would be arranged in numerical order from highest to lowest, or vice versa.

Median Used in Average Length of Stay

The list in Table 10.4 includes the LOS of fifteen discharged patients.

These numbers placed in order from highest to lowest are: 28, 21, 9, 8, 5, 5, 4, 4, 4, 4, 3, 2, 2, 2, and 1. The midpoint falls at 4. Note that, regardless of value, 50 percent of the total numbers fall above this point and 50 percent fall below. The median provides a more revealing representation of the ALOS when one or a few long-stay patients would otherwise distort the arithmetic mean. The median is not sensitive to outliers as is the mean. However, one disadvantage of using the median is that manual computation is much more time-consuming than computation of the mean. Moreover, it would be impractical with a large number of discharged patients. If the statistical computation is manual, it would be better to use the first option above. However, if the statistical computation is computerized, it would be better to use the second option.

According to table 10.4, patients on the clinical medicine service stayed 28, 8, 5, 5, 4, 4 and 2 days for a total of 56 days. Using the formula, the ALOS for medicine patients is 8.0 days ($\frac{56}{7}$). The median, or midpoint, is 5. One patient had a long stay of 28 days. If that patient is removed from the calculation, the ALOS for medicine patients would be 4.7 days. In this case, the median would be a better choice to show the ALOS for these patients.

Mode

Mode is the third measure of central tendency and is the value that occurs most frequently in the data. In this sense, it is the value that is most typical. Its advantage is that it is the simplest of the measures of central tendency because it does not require any calculations. Referring to the first example above, the mode would be three because three is the most frequent value in the set.

Table 10.4.   LOS of Fifteen Discharged Patients

Name	Age	Clinical Service	Admission Date	Length of Stay
Adams	23	Medicine	6/01	4
Baldridge	68	Medicine	5/28	8
Carpenter	62	Medicine	6/01	4
Davis	12	Medicine	5/08	28
Edison	56	Surgery	6/01	4
Faison	87	Medicine	5/31	5
Garsten	19	Obstetrics	6/03	2
Halstead	35	Obstetrics	6/01	4
Isben	67	Medicine	6/03	2
Jackson	54	Surgery	5/15	21
Kaspan	29	Obstetrics	6/03	2
Lorenzo	78	Medicine	5/31	5
Martin	42	Obstetrics	6/02	3
Nasbin	32	Obstetrics	6/04	1
Ottoperin	98	Surgery	5/27	9
Totals				**102**

While the mode is simple to use, there are disadvantages to using it. In the case of a small number of values, each value could occur only once and there will be no mode. Or, two values may be more common than others and you could have two or more modes.

Handy Tip: The mode does not have to be numerical. If you ask every person in your class what his or her favorite food is and tally the answers, you will most likely find a mode.

Example: Add another patient's LOS of 35 to the LOS example previously used on page 175 to illustrate the mean and the median. The values would now total 56 (1 + 2 + 3 + 3 + 3 + 4 + 5 + 35). Divide 56 by the number of values involved (8) to calculate the mean of 7, or $\frac{56}{8} = 7$.

The median would be calculated as follows:

1

2

3

$3 \leftarrow \text{median}\left(3 + 3 = \frac{6}{2} = 3\right)$

3

4

5

35

The median is 3, and the mode remains at 3.

This example shows that the median and the mode can be unaffected by extreme values.

The mode is rarely used as a sole descriptive measure of central tendency because it may not be unique; there may be two or more modes. These are called bimodal (two modes) or multimodal (several modes) distributions.

Example: The following represents a collection of values of lengths of stay:

1

1

1

2

2

3

3

3

4

5

5

5

7

9

In this group of patients, the mode for the LOS is 1, 3, and 5. The mode is the score that occurs most frequently; in this example, it occurred three times in 1, 3, and 5.

The choice of a measure of central tendency depends on the number of values and the nature of their distribution. Occasionally the mean, median, and mode are identical. For statistical analyses, however, the mean is preferable, whenever possible, because it includes information from all observations. However, if the series of values contains a few that are unusually high or low, the median may represent the series better than the mean. The mode is often used in samples where the most typical value is preferred.

Exercise 10.2

Complete the following exercises.

1. Fourteen patients have the following LOS: 1, 4, 4, 2, 5, 16, 3, 3, 1, 6, 4, 5, 7, and 2. Compute the mean, median, and mode.

2. A student's scores on ten 10-point class quizzes include a 6, a 7, a 4, five 9s, an 8, and a 10. The student claims that her average grade on quizzes is 9 because most of her scores are 9s. Is this correct? Explain.

3. Last month, ten patients between the ages of 11 and 13 were seen in their pediatrician's clinic. Their heights were recorded as 50, 56, 59, 51, 53, 51, 50, 52, 54 and 51 inches. Determine the mean, median, and mode.

4. An HIM supervisor timed his staff for eight hours during the workday to determine the average number of inpatient records coded in one hour. Using the findings listed below, what were the mean, median, and mode for each coder? What was the overall mean, median, and mode for the coding section?

Community Hospital
HIM Department
Number of Records Coded

Coder A		Coder B		Coder C		Coder D	
Hour 1	4	Hour 1	4	Hour 1	6	Hour 1	5
Hour 2	3	Hour 2	4	Hour 2	5	Hour 2	5
Hour 3	5	Hour 3	5	Hour 3	2	Hour 3	4
Hour 4	2	Hour 4	2	Hour 4	3	Hour 4	4
Hour 5	6	Hour 5	3	Hour 5	5	Hour 5	3
Hour 6	5	Hour 6	5	Hour 6	5	Hour 6	3
Hour 7	3	Hour 7	5	Hour 7	3	Hour 7	4
Hour 8	3	Hour 8	3	Hour 8	2	Hour 8	2

Answers:

Coder A:

Coder B:

Coder C:

Coder D:

Overall:

Measures of Variation

Measures of central tendency are not the only statistics used to summarize a frequency distribution. The facility also may want to consider the spread of the distribution, or the measure of variation. The measure of variation shows how widely the observations are spread out around the measure of central tendency. The mean gives a measure of central tendency of a list of numbers but tells nothing about the spread of the numbers in the list.

Example: Review the following three groups:

Group A	3	5	6	3	3
Group B	4	4	4	4	4
Group C	10	1	0	0	9

Each of these groups has a mean of 4 ($\frac{20}{5}$), and yet it is clear that the amount of dispersion or variation within the groups is different. The measures of spread increase with greater variation in the frequency distribution. The spread is equal to zero when there is no variation, for example, when all the values in a frequency distribution are the same, as shown in group B.

Variability

Variability refers to the difference between each score and every other score. For example, if there are 100 scores, you would have to compute the difference between the first score and each of the 99 other scores, and then compute the difference between the second score and each of the 98 remaining scores, and so on. There would be 4,950 differences in all. A more feasible approach, which serves the purpose equally well, is to define the differences or deviations for a single score in terms of how far it is from the average or the mean.

Range

The **range** is the simplest measure of spread. It indicates the difference between the largest and smallest values in a frequency distribution. In reviewing the three groups in the previous section on variability, the largest number in group A is 6 and the smallest is 3, a difference of 3. In group B, the difference is 0, and in group C, the difference is 10. Therefore, the range for group A is 3, the range for group B is 0, and the range for group C is 10.

Range has the advantage of being easy to compute. It is the simplest, order-based measure of spread, but it is far from optimal as a measure of variability for two reasons. First, as the sample size increases, the range also tends to increase. Second, it is obviously affected by extreme values that are very different from other values in the data.

Exercise 10.3

Complete the following exercises.

1. Fourteen patients have the following LOS: 2, 3, 3, 1, 4, 18, 3, 2, 1, 5, 4, 3, 6, 1. What is the range of this distribution of numbers?

2. Find the range in the following sets:
   a. 4, 3, 7, 15, 6, 8
   b. 0, –1, 8, 15, –4, 7.65
   c. 85, 91, 127, 76, 42, 47

3. The range in a frequency distribution is 22. If the lowest value is 3, what is the highest value?

4. The range in a frequency distribution is 54. If the highest value is 107, what is the lowest value?

5. A group of women seen at a diabetes clinic weighed 145, 127, 209, 216, 154, 165, 174, and 227 pounds. What is the range?

Because the range is determined by the two extremes only, a preferable measure of variability would include the distribution of all the values, not just those at the extremes. More informative measures of variation are variance and standard deviation.

Variance

The **variance** of a frequency distribution is the average of the standard deviations from the mean. The symbol s^2 is used to show the variance of a sample. "The variance of a distribution is larger when the observations are widely spread" (Johns 2007, 438). The formula for calculating the variance is:

$$s^2 = \frac{(X_1 - \bar{X})^2 + (X_2 - \bar{X})^2 + (X_3 - \bar{X})^2 \ and \ so \ on}{N - 1}$$

Or you could use the notation of

$$s^2 = \frac{\Sigma(X - \bar{X})^2}{N - 1}$$

To calculate the variance, first determine the mean. Then, the squared deviations of the mean are calculated by subtracting the mean of the frequency distribution from each value in the distribution. The difference between the two values is squared $(X - \overline{X})^2$. The squared differences are summed and divided by $N - 1$.

S^2 = variance

Σ = sum

X = value of a measure or observation

$\overline{X}$ = mean

N = number of values or observations

$N - 1$ is used in the denominator instead of N to adjust for the fact that the mean of the sample is used as an estimate of the mean of the underlying population.

The more the values in a distribution are unequal, the greater the variance and standard deviation. On page 179, the variance in group B equals 0 because all the values are the same. Measures of variation equal zero when there is no variation.

Example: To calculate the variance using the previous data, a sample of fourteen patients has the following LOS: 2, 3, 3, 1, 4, 18, 3, 2, 1, 5, 4, 3, 6, 1. In the next computation, $\overline{X}$ is the actual LOS per patient. The mean LOS is calculated as follows:

$$\frac{56}{14} = 4 \text{ days}$$

The order of this computation is as follows:

1. Subtract the mean from each score (column 3).

2. Square each result (column 4).

3. Add columns 3 and 4.

4. Divide column 4 by $(N - 1)$.

The variance is computed as follows:

$$s^2 = \frac{(2-4)^2 + (3-4)^2 + (3-4)^2 + (1-4)^2 + (4-4)^2 \, and \, so \, on}{(14-1)} = \frac{240}{13} = 18.46$$

Column 1	Column 2	Column 3	Column 4
		LOS – Mean (4)	(LOS – Mean)²
Patient	Length of Stay	$(X - \bar{X})$	$(X - \bar{X})^2$
1	2	–2	4
2	3	–1	1
3	3	–1	1
4	1	–3	9
5	4	0	0
6	18	14	196
7	3	–1	1
8	2	–2	4
9	1	–3	9
10	5	1	1
11	4	0	0
12	3	–1	1
13	6	2	4
14	1	–3	9
Total	**56**	**0**	**240**

In this example, the size of the variance is influenced by the one LOS of 18 days. The more the values in a distribution are unequal, the greater the variance and standard deviation.

Handy Tip: The sum of the deviations from the mean is always equal to zero. Therefore, by squaring the differences from the mean, the negative and positive deviations do not cancel each other out. When they are squared, negative as well as positive values become positive.

Standard Deviation

The **standard deviation** is the square root of the variance. As such, it can be more easily interpreted as a measure of variation. If the SD is small, there is less dispersion around the mean. If the SD is large, there is greater dispersion around the mean.

Handy Tip: The square root of a number is that number whose square is the number. The square of a number is that number multiplied by itself. For example, the square root of 9 is 3 (3 × 3 = 9).

To understand this concept, it is helpful to learn about what mathematicians call normal distribution of data. A **normal distribution of data** means that most of the values in a set of data are close to the "average" and relatively few values tend to one extreme or the other, creating a bell-shaped curve.

The SD is a statistic that tells how closely all the observations are clustered around the mean in a set of data. When the examples are closely gathered and the bell-shaped curve is steep, the SD is small. When the examples are spread apart and the bell-shaped curve is relatively flat, the SD is relatively large.

Therefore, normal distribution means that if the variable on every person in the population were measured, the frequency distribution would display a normal pattern, with most of the **measurements** near the center of the frequency. It also would be possible to accurately describe the population, with respect to a variable, by calculating the mean, variance, and SD of the values.

Example: Computing the value of a standard deviation can be complicated. Figure 10.1 shows an example of a normal distribution. The center, or mean, is at 6. The SD in this example is 2.45. This means that about 68 percent of the observations in the frequency distribution fall within 2.45 standard deviation of 6 (6 ± 2.45). Thus, 68 percent fall between 3.55 and 8.45; 95 percent fall between 1.1 and 10.9; and 99.7 percent fall between −1.35 and 13.35.

The formula for calculating standard deviation is:

$$SD = \sqrt{\frac{\sum(X - \bar{X})^2}{(N-1)}}$$

Figure 10.1.   Example of Normal Distribution

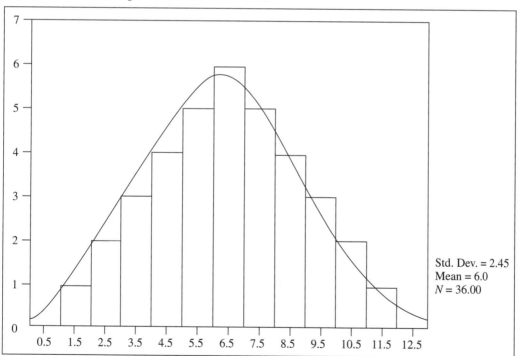

Std. Dev. = 2.45
Mean = 6.0
N = 36.00

Example: Continuing with the LOS example on page 181, the mean is 4 and the variance is 18.46. Thus, the SD is 4.3 (the square root of 18.46 = 4.30).

This means that ±1 SD contains values ranging from –0.3 to 8.3 (to get these figures add 1 SD to the mean of 4 so ±1 SD = 4 – 4.3 to 4 + 4.3 = –0.3 to 8.3).

±2 SD includes values ranging from –4.6 to 12.6 (to get these figures add 2 SD to the mean of 4 so ±2 SD = –0.3 + 4.3 to 4.3 + 8.3 = –4.6 to 12.6).

And ±3 SD includes all values ranging from –8.9 to 16.9.

Figure 10.2 shows a **graph** of standard deviation of the LOS example.

Example: In evaluating the LOS data, one can conclude that 13 out of 14 (92.9%) LOS fell within ±1 SD from the mean. The remaining value, 18, falls outside the ±3 SD from the mean and is called an outlier.

It should be noted that the distribution above is not a normal distribution. As stated earlier, in a normal distribution, one SD in both directions from the mean contains 68.3 percent of all values. In this data set, approximately 93 percent of the scores fall between ±1 SD from the mean. Visual inspection of the data in the LOS example reveals a fairly homogeneous data set despite the large SD. This emphasizes the importance of visual inspection of the data set when making decisions based on statistical calculations.

Figure 10.2.   Example of Standard Deviation

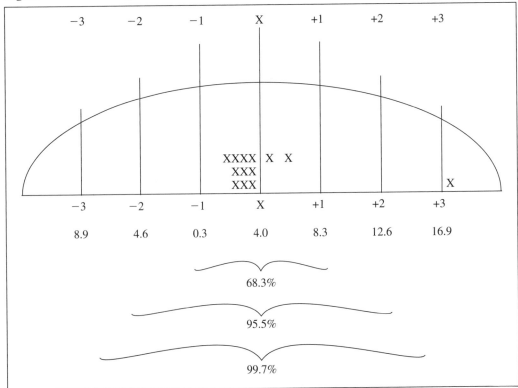

Source: Huffman

Exercise 10.4

The following sample report from a cancer registry shows the SDs of weights for twenty males with adenocarcinoma of the rectum. Validate the calculations used in the report.

Weights of Males with Adenocarcinoma of Rectum

Patient	Weight lbs. (X)	($X - \bar{X}$)	($X - \bar{X}$)^2
1	142	−30	900
2	148	−24	576
3	151	−21	441
4	155	−17	289
5	155	−17	289
6	158	−14	196
7	164	−8	64
8	165	−7	49
9	170	−2	4
10	173	1	1
11	175	3	9
12	175	3	9
13	175	3	9
14	183	11	121
15	185	13	169
16	186	14	196
17	189	17	289
18	193	21	441
19	198	26	676
20	200	28	784
Total No. of Patients	**20**	**3,440**	**0**	**5,512**

*SD = 17.0; $s^2 = \frac{5,512}{19} = 290.1$; mean = 172; and $N - 1 = 19$

Not all distributions are symmetrical or have the usual bell-shaped curve. Some curves are skewed; that is, their numbers do not fall in the middle but, rather, on one end of the curve. **Skewness** is the horizontal stretching of a frequency distribution to one side or the other so that one tail is longer than the other. The direction of skewness is on the side of the long tail. Thus, if the longer tail is on the right, the curve is skewed to the right. If the longer tail is on the left, the curve is skewed to the left. (See figures 10.3 and 10.4.)

Figure 10.3.   Example of a Curve Skewed to the Right (Positive Skew)

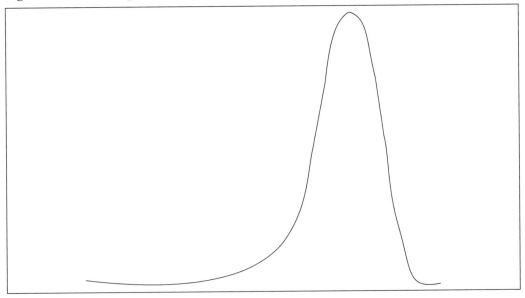

Figure 10.4.   Example of a Curve Skewed to the Left (Negative Skew)

An example of skewness may occur in lengths of stay when one or more of a group of patients has an unusually long LOS. An unusually long LOS would raise the mean and thus result in a positive skewness.

Other Curves

Although less common than the normal, positive, and negative skewed curves, you may come across other types of curves in the graphical representation of data. Some examples

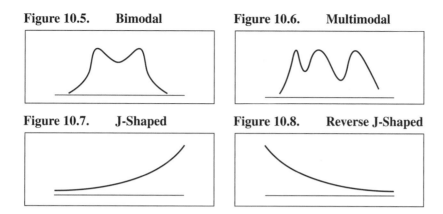

Figure 10.5.   Bimodal

Figure 10.6.   Multimodal

Figure 10.7.   J-Shaped

Figure 10.8.   Reverse J-Shaped

of the other types of curves include a bimodal distribution, multimodal distribution, a J-shaped curve, and a reverse J-shaped curve, which are shown in figures 10.5–10.8.

Correlation

Correlation (represented by r) measures the extent of a linear relationship between two variables and can be described as strong, moderate, or weak, and positive or negative. A positive relationship between two variables is direct, and a negative relationship is inverse. An example of a direct relationship is height and weight; generally the taller a person is, the more he or she weighs. An example of an inverse relationship could be when the number of prescriptions for hormone replacement therapy written by physicians goes down, the prescriptions for antidepressants goes up. It is important to remember that correlation does not imply causation; in other words, just because two variables are highly correlated does not mean that one *causes* the other.

The value for correlation will always be between −1 and +1. A correlation of 0 means there is no relationship between the variables. The closer r is to −1 or +1, the stronger the relationship, and the closer r is to 0 the weaker the relationship. −1 implies a perfect negative (inverse) relationship and +1 implies a perfect positive (direct) relationship. Chapter 11 shows three sample scatter diagrams showing a positive and negative relationship, and one showing no relationship.

To compute the correlation r between values x and y, use the formula:

$$r = \frac{\sum xy - \dfrac{\sum x \sum y}{n}}{\sqrt{\left(\sum x^2 - \dfrac{(\sum x)^2}{n}\right)\left(\sum y^2 - \dfrac{(\sum y)^2}{n}\right)}}$$

Where:

$\sum x$ is the sum of all the x values.

$\sum y$ is the sum of all the y values.

$\sum xy$ is the sum of all the x values multiplied by the y values.

$\sum x^2$ is the sum of the squares of all x values.

$\sum y^2$ is the sum of the squares of all y values.

n is the number of subjects in the group.

Example: In this example, X = the number of phone calls per week to make an appointment to see a new psychologist; Y = the number of actual visits to the psychologist plus any walk-ins.

Raw Values

x	y
5	1
6	4
9	8
11	9
14	14
15	16
21	18
$\bar{x} = 11.57$	$\bar{y} = 10$
$\Sigma x = 81$	$\Sigma y = 70$
$\Sigma x^2 = 1,125$	$\Sigma y^2 = 938$
$(\Sigma x)^2 = 6,561$	$(\Sigma y)^2 = 4,900$
$n = 7$	$n = 7$

$$\Sigma xy = 1,014$$

In this example, the values for Σx, Σy, Σx^2, Σy^2, $(\Sigma x)^2$, $(\Sigma y)^2$ and Σxy are computed as follows:

$\Sigma x = (5 + 6 + 9 + 11 + 14 + 15 + 21)$
$\Sigma x = 81$

$\Sigma y = (1 + 4 + 8 + 9 + 14 + 16 + 18)$
$\Sigma y = 70$

$\Sigma x^2 = (5^2 + 6^2 + 9^2 + 11^2 + 14^2 + 15^2 + 21^2)$
$\Sigma x^2 = 1,125$

$\Sigma y^2 = (1^2 + 4^2 + 8^2 + 9^2 + 14^2 + 16^2 + 18^2)$
$\Sigma y^2 = 938$

$\Sigma (x)^2 = (81)^2$
$\Sigma (x)^2 = 6,561$

$\Sigma (y)^2 = (70)^2$
$\Sigma (y)^2 = 4,900$

$\Sigma xy = (5 \times 1) + (6 \times 4) + (9 \times 8)\,(11 \times 9) + (14 \times 14) + (15 \times 16) + (21 \times 18)$
$\Sigma xy = 1,014$

Next, plug these values into the formula for r.

$$r = \frac{1,014 - \dfrac{(81)(70)}{7}}{\sqrt{\left(1,125 - \dfrac{6,561}{7}\right)\left(938 - \dfrac{4,900}{7}\right)}}$$

$$r = \frac{1,014 - 810}{\sqrt{(1,125 - 937.29)(938 - 700)}}$$

$$r = \frac{204}{\sqrt{(187.71)(238)}}$$

$$r = .97$$

In this example, $r = .97$ is a very strong positive correlation. Although causation cannot be implied, it can still be said that there is a strong direct relationship between x and y. In this case, there is a very strong correlation between the number of appointments made and the number of actual visits made with the psychologist.

Calculating the correlation can be a lengthy process, especially if there are a large number of subjects. Therefore, after learning how to do the process by hand, it is best to use computer software or a calculator that is capable of computing r from keying in the values of x and y; in this way, your answer will be more accurate.

Calculations for variance, standard deviation, and correlation are not usually part of the health information technician's day-to-day activities; however, it is important to be familiar with these concepts. For example, you may pick up a journal article or listen to a speaker who is discussing these calculations and an understanding of them may be necessary in order to communicate this information with others.

Chapter 10 Test

1. Your medical terminology instructor listed the following grades for the class out of a 75-point test:

   33, 34, 43, 45, 45, 54, 55, 59, 60, 62, 64, 66, 67, 68, 67, 68, 68, 69, 70, 70

   a. Find the 90th percentile.
   b. Your score was 59, what is your percentile?

2. From the following list of number of discharges each day in September, compute the mean, median, mode, and range. Round the mean and median to one decimal point

Community Hospital
Number of Discharge Days
September 20XX

Day	No. of Discharges	Day	No. of Discharges	Day	No. of Discharges
1	27	11	36	21	53
2	22	12	75	22	59
3	35	13	65	23	54
4	63	14	84	24	52
5	42	15	37	25	32
6	55	16	38	26	64
7	2	17	62	27	67
8	65	18	65	28	69
9	32	19	48	29	58
10	35	20	55	30	55

(continued on next page)

Chapter 10 Test (continued)

3. Use the following dates to compute the ALOS and median LOS and range. The discharge date is July 2nd (non-leap year). Round the ALOS to one decimal place.

Admission Date	LOS
2-10	February = 18; March = 31; April = 30; May = 31; June = 30; July = 2; Total = 142
3-15	March = 16; April = 30; May = 31; June = 30; July = 2; Total = 109
3-1	March = 30; April = 30; May = 31; June = 30; July = 2; Total = 123
5-6	May = 25; June = 30; July = 2; Total = 57
2-26	February = 2; March = 31; April = 30; May = 31; June = 30; July = 2; Total = 126
4-15	April = 15; May = 31; June = 30; July = 2; Total = 78
5-5	May = 26; June = 30; July = 2; Total = 58
6-17	June = 13; July = 2; Total = 15
6-29	June = 1; July = 2; Total = 3
5-18	May = 13; June = 30; July = 2; Total = 45
3-12	March = 19; April = 30; May = 31; June = 30; July = 2; Total = 112
7-1	July 2; Total = 1
2-8	February = 20; March = 31; April = 30; May = 31; June = 30; July = 2; Total = 144
5-3	May = 28; June = 30; July = 2; Total = 60
1-2	January = 29; February = 28; March = 31; April = 30; May = 31; June = 30; July = 2; Total = 181
3-6	March = 25; April = 30; May = 31; June = 30; July = 2; Total = 118
4-1	April = 29; May = 31; June = 30; July = 2; Total = 92
1-10	January = 21; February = 2; March = 31; April = 30; May = 31; June = 30; July = 2; Total = 173
3-1	March = 30; April = 30; May = 31; June = 30; July = 2; Total = 123

4. When two variables are correlated, it means that one is the cause of the other. True or False?

Chapter 10 Test (continued)

5. The table below shows the LOS for a sample of eleven discharged patients. Using the data in the table, calculate the mean, range, variance, and standard deviation, and then answer questions e and f. Round the variance and standard deviation to one decimal place

   a. Mean
   b. Range
   c. Variance
   d. Standard deviation
   e. What value is affecting the mean and SD of this distribution?
   f. Does the mean adequately represent this distribution? If not, what would be a better measure of central tendency for this data set?

Patient	Length of Stay	LOS – Mean (5) $(X - \bar{X})$	(LOS – Mean)^2 $(X - \bar{X})^2$
1	1		
2	3		
3	5		
4	3		
5	2		
6	29		
7	3		
8	4		
9	2		
10	1		
11	2		

Chapter 11
Presentation of Data

Objectives

At the conclusion of this chapter, you should be able to:

- Discuss categorical data: nominal, ordinal, interval, and ratio

- Differentiate between discrete data and continuous data

- Describe and differentiate between tables and the following graphs: bar graphs, pie charts, line graphs, histograms, frequency polygons, pictograms, and scatter diagrams

- Create tables and graphs to display statistical information

- Understand the basic elements in preparing a report

Types of Data

A set of raw data may not necessarily provide a user (such as an administrator, a physician, or an HIM professional) with information that can be easily interpreted. Descriptive statistics are the most common type of statistics that the health information technician will encounter or be responsible for producing. Descriptive statistics describe populations, which can refer to patients, medical services, nursing units, or hospital departments. As mentioned in Chapter 10, these statistics provide an overview of the general features of a set of data. The statistics can assume a number of different forms, the most common being tables and graphs. However, before choosing the appropriate method for displaying a set of data, it is important to determine whether the data are categorical or numerical.

Categorical Data

There are four types or **scales of measurement** of **categorical data**: nominal, ordinal, ratio, and interval. Ratio and interval data are considered metric variables. Metric variables are numeric variables that answer questions of how much or how many.

Nominal Data

Nominal data are the lowest level of measurement. The word *nominal* means "pertaining to a name." In the nominal scale, observations are organized into categories in which there is no recognition of order. Examples of nominal data include true/false, male/female, types of insurance carriers, or patient occupations. Often numbers are used to represent categories. For example, a male may be listed as 1 and a female as 2; or persons may be grouped according to blood type, where 1 represents type A; 2, type B; 3, type AB; and 4, type O. The sequence of the values is not important. The numbers simply serve as labels for some piece of information and are used for convenience only.

Averages cannot be computed on nominal-level data. For example, an average blood type of 2.3 for a given population is meaningless. Instead of calculating the mean for nominal data, the proportion (or "how many") that falls into each category is reported. The following types of healthcare payment categories are an example of nominal data.

Payment Categories

1 Medicare

2 Medicaid

3 Blue Cross

4 Other Commercial Insurance

5 Self-pay

6 Other

Ordinal Data

Ordinal data are types of data where the values are in ordered categories. The word *ordinal* means "to put something in order." On the ordinal scale, only the order of the numbers is meaningful, not the numbers themselves. This is because the intervals or distances between categories are not necessarily equal. For example, head injuries may be classified according to level of severity, where 4 is fatal; 3, severe; 2, moderate; and 1, minor.

A natural order exists among the groupings, with the largest number representing the most serious level of injury. However, the order could be reversed; there is no hard-and-fast rule. There is no reason why 1 could not represent the fatal injury and 4, the minor injury. In addition, the distance between a fatal and a severe injury may not necessarily be the same as the distance between a moderate and a minor injury. The following list shows how this works in a classification of brain injury.

1   Minor

2   Moderate

3   Severe

4   Fatal

Another good example of ordinal data is the Likert scale used in many surveys: 1 = strongly disagree; 2 = disagree; 3 = neutral; 4 = agree; 5 = strongly agree. In this example, there is a natural order 1 through 5; however, 1 could just as easily be strongly agree and 5, strongly disagree.

Interval Data

Interval data include units of equal size, such as intelligence quotient (IQ) results. There is no zero point. An example is temperature in Fahrenheit degrees. The intervals between the values are the same. The most important characteristic is that the intervals between values are equal.

Another example of interval scale is time. Time is measured in terms of 24 hours in a day. The time between each hour is the same. For example, there are 60 minutes between 1:00 a.m. and 2:00 a.m. and between 5:00 p.m. and 6:00 p.m.

Ratio Data

Ratio data or scale is the highest level of measurement. On the ratio scale, there is a defined unit of measure, a real zero point, and the intervals between successive values are equal. Ratio data may be displayed by units of equal size placed on a scale starting with zero and thus can be manipulated mathematically, such as 0, 5, 10, 15, and 20.

Example: An example of the ratio scale is age. The difference between two years would be the same (the difference between age 1 and 2 is 1 year; the difference between age 55 and 56 is one year, and so on). There is a "zero point" in that zero would mean an absence of age or birth; and someone who is 100 years old is twice as old as someone who is 50 years old.

Exercise 11.1

Review the following table and answer the questions below.

**Community Hospital
Discharges by Gender
Annual Statistics 20XX**

Males	1,203
Females	1,235

1. What example of scales of measurement is depicted in the table?

2. Your health information instructor reported that on the last test given, five students received an A, ten received a B, three received a C, one received a D, and no one received an F. What example of scales of measurement was given?

3. Is it accurate to state that a temperature of 80 degrees F is twice as hot as 40 degrees F?

4. If a physician's office saw 50 patients yesterday and 100 patients today, is it correct to state that twice as many patients were seen today as yesterday?

5. A physician's clinic conducted a survey to determine the level of patient satisfaction with various departments in the clinic. What type of scale is the following survey item?

> The information clerk at the clinic gave me the correct directions to find the department I was looking for.
>
> Please answer this question on a scale from 1 to 5 where 1 = strongly disagree and 5 = strongly agree.

6. A physician on your staff asked you to help her collect information on the effects of drinking alcohol on pregnancy and the birth weight of babies. You were asked to collect the following information.

   Did the mothers drink alcohol during pregnancy (yes or no)

   Birth weight of the baby

   Apgar score at 1 minute

   Apgar score at 5 minutes

   The scales of these variables would be:
   a. nominal, ordinal, interval and ratio
   b. nominal, ratio, ordinal, ordinal
   c. ordinal, nominal, ratio, interval
   d. ratio, ordinal, interval, nominal

Numerical Data

There are two types of numerical statistical data: discrete data and continuous data.

Discrete Data

Discrete data are finite numbers. That is, they can have only specified values. The number of children in a family is an example of discrete data. A family can have two or three children but cannot have 2.25 or 3.5 children. The numbers represent actual measurable quantities rather than labels.

Other examples of discrete data include the number of motor vehicle accidents in a particular community, the number of times a woman has given birth, the number of new cases of cancer in your state within the past five years, and the number of beds available in your hospital.

In discrete data, a natural order exists among the possible data values. In the example of the number of times a woman has given birth, a larger number indicates that she has had more children; the difference between one and two births is the same as the difference between four and five; and the number of births is restricted to whole numbers (a woman cannot give birth 2.3 times). For the most part, measurements on the nominal and ordinal scales are discrete.

Continuous Data

Continuous data represent measurable quantities but are not restricted to certain specified values. A variable that is continuous can take on a fractional value. For example, a patient's temperature may be 102.6° F. Another example is height. One could say that someone is approximately 6 feet tall, refine it to 5 feet 10 inches, and refine it still further to 5 feet $10\frac{1}{2}$ inches. Age is yet another example. You may have been 20 years old on your last birthday, but now you are 20 plus some part of another year.

The only limiting factor for a continuous observation is the degree of accuracy with which it can be measured. For analysis, continuous data often are converted to a range that acts as a category. For example, age can be categorized in ranges (0–20, 21–40, and so on). Measurements on the interval and ratio scales can be grouped; interval and ratio variables are continuous.

Data Display

Data display is critical to data analysis because it reveals patterns and behaviors. When preparing a statistical report, the user must define its objectives and scope:

- What information is needed?
- What information is available?
- Are the data collected routinely by the facility, or must additional data be collected?

If the purpose requires frequencies, percentages, or relationships among variables, the data may be presented in the form of a table or a graph. Basically, statistical tables are used for summarizing data; they simply list values into rows and columns and do not easily capture the audience's attention. On the other hand, graphs and charts can present data for quick visualization of relationships.

Tables

A **table** is an orderly arrangement of values that groups data into rows and columns. Almost any type of quantitative information can be grouped into tables. Columns allow you to read data up and down, and rows allow you to read data across. The columns and rows should be labeled. Many word-processing, spreadsheet, and database software programs offer assistance in the creation of tables. In table 11.1, variables arranged in columns across the page identify the individual patient name, age, clinical service, and length of stay. Each row represents one patient.

There are a number of advantages to using tables, including:

- More information can be presented.
- Exact values can be read to retain precision.
- Supportive details can be provided.
- Less work and fewer costs are required in the preparation.
- Flexibility is maintained without distortion of data.
- There also are many advantages to using graphs, including:
  — They get the audience's attention.
  — They are easy to understand.
  — They bring out hidden facts.
  — They vividly display trends or comparisons.
  — A picture is worth a thousand words.

Table 11.1.   Community Medical Center Analysis Showing Patients Discharged 12/1/20XX

Name	Age	Clinical Service	Length of Stay
Smith	5	Surgical	1
Valdez	22	Obstetrical	1
Chu	26	Obstetrical	2
MacDuff	18	Obstetrical	3
Johnson	10	Surgical	7
O'Brien	80	Surgical	8
Lewandowski	35	Surgical	11
Jones	52	Medical	15
Shultz	69	Medical	37
Martini	49	Medical	42

Source: Community Medical Center

The essential components of a table include:

- Title: The title must explain as simply as possible what is contained in the table. The title should answer the questions:
  — What are the data? For example, are these percentages; frequencies?
  — Who? Who is the table about? For instance, are these males or females; a certain service; a type of disease?
  — Where? For example, is this your hospital; the U.S.; or your state?
  — When? What is the time period?
- Stub heading: The title or heading of the first column
- Column headings: The headings or titles for the columns
- Stubs: The categories (the left-hand column of a table)
- Cells: The information formed by intersecting columns and rows
- Source footnote: The source for any factual data should be identified in a footnote.

Table 11.2 illustrates the essential components of a table.

Table 11.2.   The Essential Components of a Table

	Title		
Stub Heading	**Column Heading**	**Column Heading**	**Column Heading**
Stub	Cell	Cell	Cell
Stub	Cell	Cell	Cell
Stub	Cell	Cell	Cell

Source: Reprinted, with permission, from SEER Program, *Self-Instructional Manual for Cancer Registrars, Book 7* (Washington, D.C.: U.S. Department of Health and Human Services, 1994, p. 23).

Table 11.3 shows a sample table with completed components.

Table 11.3.   Lung Cancer by Age and Gender at Community Hospital 20XX

Community Hospital Lung Cancer by Age and Gender Annual Statistics 20XX		
Age, years	**Male**	**Female**
≤ 30	1	0
31–40	2	1
41–50	2	1
51–60	10	10
61–70	42	44
71 +	29	27
Totals	**86**	**83**

Although these rules are important in the construction of tables, it is more important to use good judgment. Check the table to be sure that it is logical and self-explanatory. Are headings specific and understandable for every column and row? Do totals add up? Is the table easy to read? Remember to present the data in a format that illustrates a specific idea.

Frequency Distribution Tables

A frequency distribution shows the values that a variable can take and the number of observations associated with each value. A variable is a characteristic or property that may take on different values. For example, third-party payers, discharge service, and admission day are examples of variables.

> **Example:** The Utilization Review Committee is interested in knowing the admission days for patients in your hospital. To construct a frequency distribution, you would list the days of the week and then enter the observations or number of patients admitted on the corresponding day of the week. Table 11.4 illustrates what this would look like.

A frequency distribution table also may show the proportion, that is, the proportion of patients admitted on any of the days. To determine this, the value is divided by the total. The total should always equal 1.00.

Table 11.5 shows the same frequency distribution as in the example in table 11.4, but with the proportion added. Notice that to arrive at the proportion, the student should divide the number of patients admitted by the total. For example, Sunday shows 20 admissions of the 132 total.

$$\frac{20}{132} = 0.15$$

Table 11.6 shows a frequency distribution table of cigarette consumption in the United States from 1900 to 2005.

Table 11.4.   Report Illustrating Sample Frequency Distribution Table

Sample Frequency Distribution for Admission Day June 20XX	
Day of the Week	**No. of Patients Admitted**
Sunday	20
Monday	29
Tuesday	28
Wednesday	12
Thursday	13
Friday	22
Saturday	8
Total	**132**

Table 11.5.   **Report Illustrating Sample Frequency Distribution with Proportion**

Sample Frequency Distribution for Admission Day June 20XX		
Day of the Week	**No. of Patients Admitted**	**Proportion**
Sunday	20	0.15
Monday	29	0.22
Tuesday	28	0.21
Wednesday	12	0.09
Thursday	13	0.10
Friday	22	0.17
Saturday	8	0.06
Total	**132**	**1.00**

Table 11.6.   **Report Illustrating Frequency Distribution**

Cigarette Consumption United States 1900–2005	
Year	**No. of Cigarettes Consumed (in billions)**
1900	2.5
1905	3.6
1910	8.6
1915	17.9
1920	44.6
1925	79.8
1930	119.3
1935	134.4
1940	181.9
1945	340.6
1950	369.8
1955	396.4
1960	484.4
1965	528.8
1970	536.5
1975	607.2
1980	631.5
1985	594.0
1990	525.0
1995	487.0
2000	430.0
2005	376.0

Source: Tobacco Outlook Report, Economic Research Service, U.S. Dept. of Agriculture. Available at http://www.infoplease.com/ipa/A0908700.html.

To display discrete or continuous data in the form of a frequency distribution table, the range of values of the observations must be broken down into a series of distinct groups that do not overlap. For example, when arranging a frequency distribution table by patient age, age ranges should not be listed as 1–10, 10–20, 20–30, 30–40, and so on because a patient could be placed in two categories if he were age 20: the 10 to 20 age range and the 20 to 30 age range. Thus, age ranges should be listed as 1–10, 11–20, 21–30, 31–40, and so on.

Summarizing the data involves setting up categories and counting the number of cases that fall into each category, thereby creating a frequency distribution. Following are some general rules for choosing the classes or categories into which the data are to be grouped and the range of each:

- Do not use fewer than five or more than fifteen categories. However, the choice depends mostly on the number of values to be grouped.

- Categories should be well defined. Choose categories that cover the smallest and largest values and do not produce gaps between categories.

- The categories should be mutually exclusive where each observation is grouped into one—and only one—category. Avoid successive classes that overlap or have common values.

- Whenever possible, make the classes cover equal ranges (or intervals) of values. These ranges also should be made up of numbers that are easy to work with.

Exercise 11.2

The table below lists the patients seen last month at Community Hospital with their age and cholesterol reading. Create a table using common age categories and these ranges for cholesterol:

Desirable ≤ 199
Borderline High 200–239
High ≥ 240

Age	Cholesterol	Age	Cholesterol	Age	Cholesterol	Age	Cholesterol
14	118	44	138	38	165	56	185
80	139	47	204	18	142	20	200
42	187	48	236	62	139	45	241
37	201	25	186	37	202	63	175
23	107	56	201	32	207	70	188
24	109	47	198	17	157	42	239
67	132	20	210	55	238	55	175
55	235	43	248	13	134	61	168
52	185	50	137	44	239	53	173
52	192	34	188	64	165	41	238
47	144	38	245	70	172	60	180
42	158	75	175	44	245	30	207
37	160	55	207	65	187	62	185
33	155	69	192	51	248	49	207
39	221	31	196	43	240	39	147
34	244	51	147	51	188	53	155
75	186	63	200	50	203	46	246
81	160	18	137	20	145	43	222
79	154	37	245	72	175	26	147
67	154	43	256	39	200	46	201
50	192	44	188	19	145	60	152
53	188	52	200	63	145	35	150
26	137	51	147	36	176	53	215
24	140	19	132	33	185	60	165
22	138	73	147	16	137	63	168

Exercise 11.3

The following table shows a frequency distribution of patients with Colon Cancer treated at Community Hospital. Compute the proportion of patients in each category.

Community Hospital
Ages of Patients with Colon Cancer
Annual Statistics 20XX

Ages	No. of Patients	Proportion
≤ 30	3	
31–40	12	
41–50	18	
51–60	60	
61–70	65	
71 +	48	

Graphs

Graphs of various types are the best means for presenting data for quick visualization of relationships.

They often supply a lesser degree of detail than tables. However, data presented in a graph can be helpful in displaying statistics in a concise manner. Graphs should be easy to read, simple in content, and correctly labeled. The presentation of data in the form of a graph is an excellent way to convey the message you want to get across. Instead of presenting an entire statistical report in a table to a group such as the medical staff or administration, you can create a graph to depict the data. Many computer software programs are available that convert data into graphic form automatically and attractively.

When creating graphs, follow these general guidelines:

- The title must relate to what the graph is displaying. Follow the same general guidelines for the title in graphs as given in tables including what are the data, who is the graph about, to whom does it refer, and the time period.

- When several variables are included on the same graph (for example, males and females), each should be identified by using a legend or key.

- Categories should be natural; that is, the vertical axis should always start with zero. The scale of values for the x-axis reads from the lowest value on the left to the highest on the right. The scale of values for the y-axis extends from the lowest value at the bottom of the graph to the highest at the top.

- Scale captions are placed on both axes to identify the values clearly. These are simply titles placed on each axis to identify the values. (See figure 11.1.)

Figure 11.1.   Scale Captions on a Graph

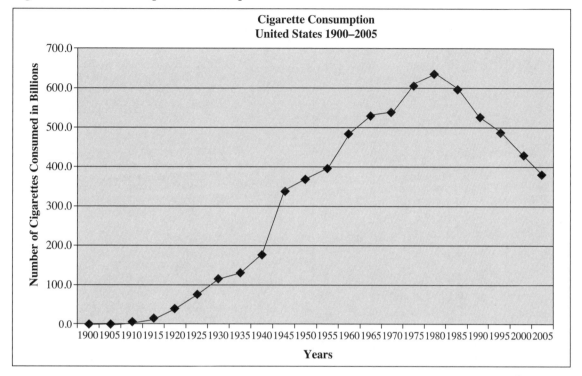

- Graphs should emphasize the horizontal. It is easier for the eye to read along the horizontal axis from left to right. Also, graphs should be greater in length than in height. A useful guideline is to follow the three-quarter-high rule, which states that the graph's height (y-axis) should be three-fourths of its length (x-axis).

- The exact reference to an outside source should be given.

Handy Tip: Selecting the most appropriate graph to accompany your data adds a great deal to the effectiveness of your presentation; however, you should avoid an overabundance of graphs. It is a good idea to produce several versions of a graph and then use the one that is most illuminating (SEER Program 1994).

Bar Graphs

Bar graphs, or **bar charts**, are appropriate for displaying categorical data. The simplest bar graph is a one-variable bar graph. In it, the various categories of observations are presented along a horizontal axis, or x-axis. (See figures 11.2 and 11.3.) The vertical axis, or y-axis, displays the frequency of the data. Data representing frequencies, proportions, or percentages of categories are often displayed using bar graphs. A grouped bar chart is used to display information from tables containing two or three variables. Figure 11.4 shows an example of a three-variable bar graph.

Figure 11.2.   Example of a One-Variable Bar Graph

**Community Hospital
Admissions by Day of the Week
January, 20XX–December, 20XX**

Source: Administrator's annual report.

Figure 11.3.   Example of a Two-Variable Bar Graph

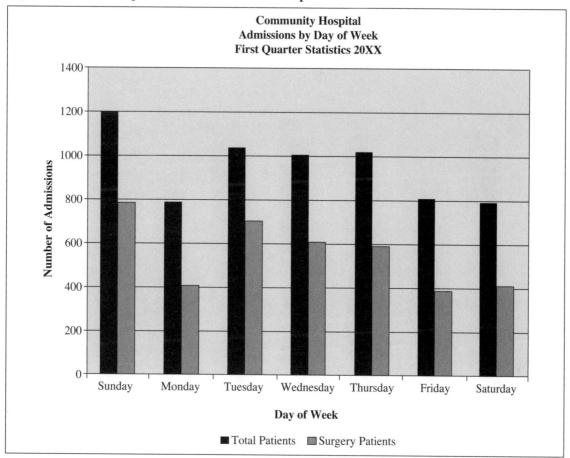

Source: Administrator's First Quarter Statistics 1/1/20XX to 3/31/20XX.

Figure 11.4.   Example of a Three-Variable Bar Graph

Pie Charts

A **pie chart**, or **pie graph**, is a method of displaying data as component parts of a whole. Use a pie chart when you want to show each category's percentage of the total. A circle is divided into sections such as wedges or slices. These represent percentages of the total (100 percent). To make a pie chart, include all the categories that make up a whole. Therefore, data must be converted into percentages unless you are working with computer software that converts your numbers into percentages. Pie chart wedges may be shaded or colored to help differentiate the sections. In addition, they can be cut out of the pie to help emphasize a percentage. Computer software programs are extremely useful when creating pie graphs. (See figures 11.5 and 11.6 for examples of pie charts.)

Figure 11.5.   **Pie Graph Showing Nosocomial Infection by Major Service Category**

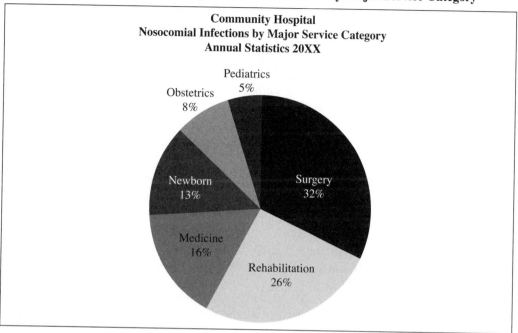

Figure 11.6.   **Pie Graph Showing Brain Injury Patients Admitted from Other Facilities**

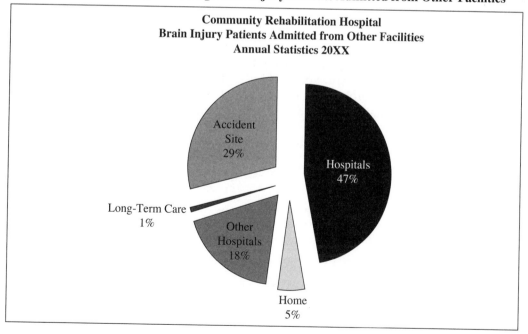

Line Graphs

A **line graph** is often used to show data over time (for example, days, weeks, months, or years). The x-axis shows the time period, and the y-axis shows the values of the variables. A line graph consists of a line connecting a series of points on an arithmetic scale. Line graphs also allow for several variables to be plotted. Line graphs are also referred to as **run charts** in the quality management field.

The x-axis depicts the units of time from left to right, and the y-axis measures the values of the variable being shown. (See figures 11.7 and 11.8 for examples of line graphs.)

Histograms

A **histogram** is a graph used to display frequency distributions for continuous numerical data (interval or ratio data). Histograms are created from frequency distribution tables. (See figures 11.9 and 11.10 for examples of histograms.) They look similar to bar graphs except that all the bars in a histogram are touching because they show the continuous nature of the distribution.

Frequency Polygon

A **frequency polygon** is similar to a histogram in that it is a graph depicting the frequency of continuous data; however, a frequency polygon is in line form instead of bar form. The advantage of a frequency polygon is that several of them can be placed on the same graph to make comparisons. A frequency polygon uses the same axes as the histogram; that is, the x-axis displays the scale of the variable and the y-axis displays the frequency. A dot is placed at the midpoint of the class interval or frequency. A line drawn from one point to the next then connects the dots. Because the x-axis represents the entire frequency distribution, the line starts at zero cases and is drawn from the last frequency to the y-axis to end with zero. (See figure 11.11.)

Pictogram

A **pictogram** is an attractive alternative type of bar graph in that it uses pictures to show the frequency of the data. For example, if you want to show the number of people with SARS treated for the past several months, you might use stick people. If you need to show exact numbers, a pictogram will probably not be a good choice for your presentation, however, they are very good at catching the attention of your audience and will give them a good idea of your data. (See figure 11.12.)

Figure 11.7.   Example of a One-Variable Line Graph

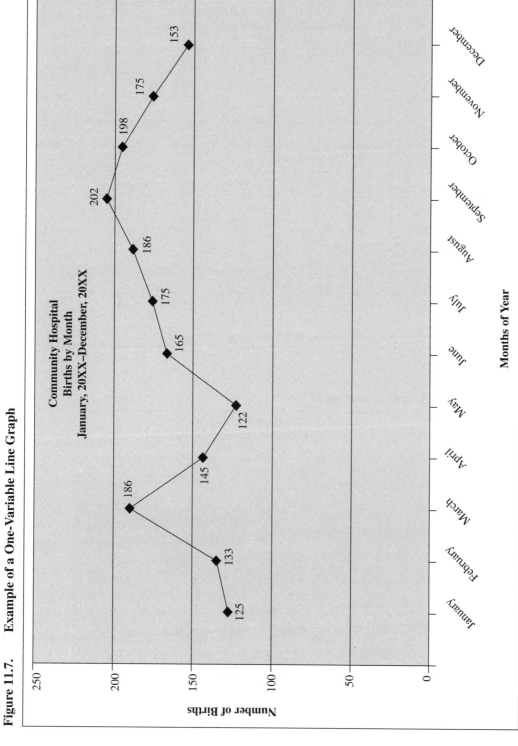

Community Hospital
Births by Month
January, 20XX–December, 20XX

Figure 11.8.   Example of a Two-Variable Line Graph

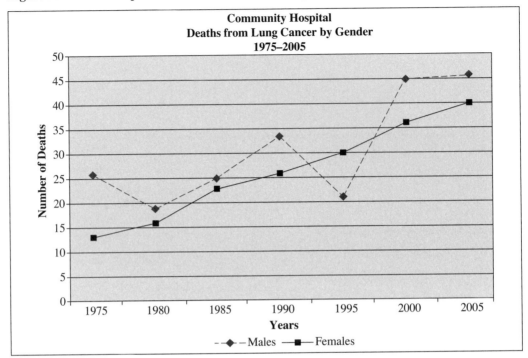

Figure 11.9.   Sample Histogram #1

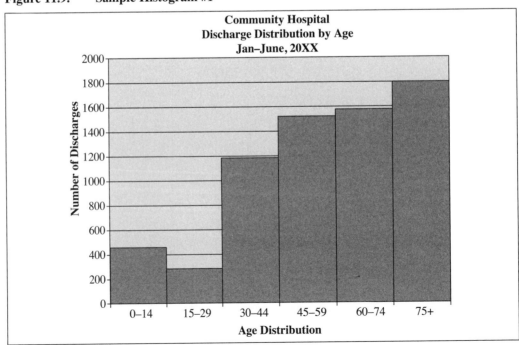

Figure 11.10.   Sample Histogram #2

Figure 11.11.   Frequency Polygon

Figure 11.12.   Sample Pictogram

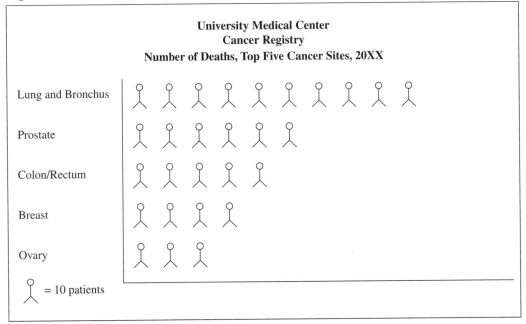

Scatter Diagram

A **scatter diagram** (also called a scattergram or scatter plot) is used to graphically show the relationship between two numerical variables. A scattergram is used to determine whether there is a correlation, or relationship, between two characteristics. Correlation implies that as one variable changes, the other also changes. This does not always mean that there is a cause-and-effect relationship between two variables because there may be other variables that could cause the change. If the two characteristics are somehow related, the pattern of points will show a tight clustering in a certain direction. The closer the points look like a line in appearance, the more the two characteristics are likely to be correlated. (See figure 11.13.)

The slope of the line in figure 11.13 is positive. Notice that small values of the x-axis correspond to small values of the y-axis and large values of the x-axis correspond to large values of the y-axis; thus, a positive linear relationship is thought to exist. The scatter diagram in figure 11.13 shows a weak correlation because the scatter points are not clustered together tightly

In contrast, figure 11.14 shows a scatter diagram with a negative linear relationship. That is, the small values of the x-axis correspond to large values of the y-axis and large values of the x-axis correspond to small values of the y-axis. Additionally, the scatter diagram in figure 11.14 shows a strong correlation because the cluster of points is tight.

Figure 11.15 illustrates a scatter diagram with no linear relationship because the scatter points are plotted randomly on the graph.

Figure 11.13.   **Sample Scatter Diagram Showing a Positive Linear Relationship**

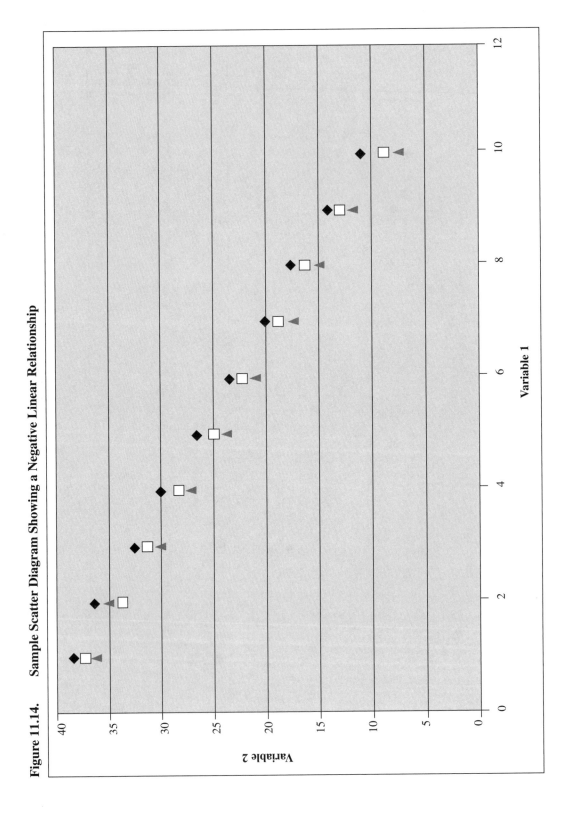

Figure 11.14.   Sample Scatter Diagram Showing a Negative Linear Relationship

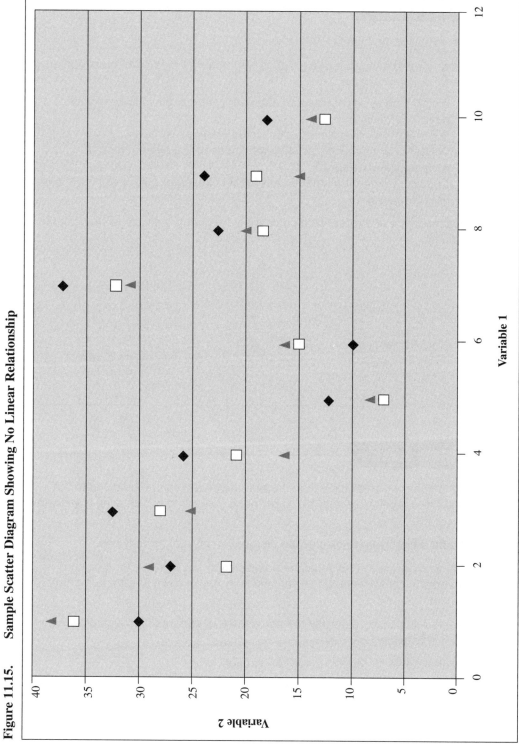

Figure 11.15. **Sample Scatter Diagram Showing No Linear Relationship**

Exercise 11.4

Complete the following exercises.

1. Indicate whether a table or a graph is the preferred method of presentation in the following situations:

   a. Distribution by site, sex, race, and time period of all cancers in your healthcare facility
   b. Survival trends over time by sex for lung cancer
   c. Display of prostate cancer stage of disease for a presentation at a professional conference
   d. Detailed treatment distribution of breast cancer for a physician on the staff of your hospital

2. Indicate which of the following categories are mutually exclusive and clearly defined.

A	B	C
0–15	≤10.0	0–10
15–30	10.1–20.0	11–20
30–45	20.1–30.0	21–30
45–60	30.1–40.0	31–40
60+	40.1–50.0	41–50
	50.1+	51+

Exercise 11.5

Analyze the report on page 219, then prepare the data displays indicated in the list below. The data displays may be neatly hand drawn or created using a software program.

1. Create a histogram to display the distribution of total days by age.

2. Create a bar graph to display the admission by day of week for Medicare patients in comparison to the admission by day of week of total number of patients.

3. Create a pie chart to display the percentage of patients discharged by major service category.

4. Create a table for length of stay distribution.

Exercise 11.5 (continued)

Administrator's Semiannual Reference Report
January–June 20XX

ALL PATIENTS, INCLUDING ONE DAY STAYS (SEPARATE)

	ADMISSIONS					DISCHARGES			
	TOTAL PTS.	% OF PTS.	SURG. PTS.	AVG. PREOP	ONE-DAY STAYS	TOTAL PTS.	% OF PTS.	AVG. LOS	ONE-DAY STAYS
SUNDAY	1,187	17.9	774	1.7	146	809	12.1	8.1	46
MONDAY	755	11.3	426	2.8	124	576	8.7	6.2	144
TUESDAY	1,085	16.3	689	2.6	135	934	14.0	7.2	115
WEDNESDAY	1,035	15.5	622	3.5	141	934	14.0	7.7	147
THURSDAY	1,024	15.3	597	2.6	139	955	14.3	7.0	132
FRIDAY	808	12.1	359	3.9	145	965	14.5	7.7	141
SATURDAY	773	11.6	417	3.0	39	1,490	22.4	6.6	144

LENGTH OF STAY DISTRIBUTION

	PATIENTS	% CASES
SAME DAY	114	1.7
1 DAY	755	11.3
2–4 DAYS	1,343	20.2
5–7 DAYS	1,555	23.3
8–14 DAYS	1,469	22.0
15–42 DAYS	1,217	18.3
43+ DAYS	210	3.2

SUMMARY BY MAJOR SERVICE CATEGORY

	PTS.	% PTS.	DISCH DAYS	% DAYS	ALOS
MEDICINE	2,005	30.0	21,052	30.6	10.5
SURGERY	1,401	21.0	7,845	11.4	5.6
GYNECOLOGY	631	9.4	6,057	8.8	9.6
OBSTETRICS	530	7.9	2,703	3.9	5.1
NEWBORN	520	7.8	2,600	3.7	5.0
PEDIATRICS	450	6.7	4,140	6.0	9.2
PSYCHIATRY	518	7.7	8,537	12.4	16.5
OTHER	608	9.1	15,798	22.9	26.0

ADMISSION BY DAY OF THE WEEK BY PAYMENT STATUS

	SELF	BLUE CROSS	COMMERCIAL	GOV'T	WORK COMP	M-CAID	M-CARE	OTHER	Total
SUNDAY	31	413	188	0	2	41	273	2	950
MONDAY	19	300	103	0	11	46	280	1	760
TUESDAY	21	400	206	1	9	45	345	2	1,029
WEDNESDAY	20	503	240	2	22	35	223	3	1,048
THURSDAY	30	365	154	0	8	24	199	1	781
FRIDAY	28	40	179	0	0	42	294	0	583
SATURDAY	30	509	246	1	6	55	301	2	1,150
TOTAL PTS.	179	2,892	1,316	4	58	288	1,915	11	
% OF PTS.	2.6	43.4	19.7	0.6	0.8	4.3	28.7	0	
TOT DIS DAYS	1,109	26,895	16,818	36	609	2,670	20,491	104	
% OF DAYS	1.6	39.1	24.4	0	0.8	4	30	0	
AVG. LOS	6.2	9.3	12.8	9.0	10.5	9.3	11	9.5	

(continued on next page)

Exercise 11.5 (continued)

SUMMARY BY AGE

	TOTAL PTS.	% OF PTS.	TOT DIS DAYS	% DAYS	ALOS
0–14	429	6.4	1,749	2.5	4.1
15–18	229	3.4	817	1.2	3.6
19–34	1,144	17.2	9,746	14.2	8.5
35–49	1,488	22.3	14,647	21.3	9.8
50–64	1,570	23.6	18,101	26.3	11.5
65+	1,803	27.1	23,672	34.4	13.1
TOTAL	6,663		68,732		10.3

Exercise 11.6

University Hospital Cancer Registry records show the following incidence of cancer in females for the past year. Construct an appropriate graph of the data.

University Hospital
Cancer Registry
Top Ten Cancer Sites—Females
20XX

Site	Number of Cases
Breast	120
Colon and rectum	42
Uterus	25
Thyroid	21
Lymphoma	20
Melanoma	19
Lung and bronchus	15
Ovary	12
Pancreas	8
Leukemia	6

Exercise 11.7

University Hospital reported the following incidence of lung and bronchus cancer patients treated at the hospital during the past 15 years. Construct a line graph of the data.

**University Hospital
Cancer Registry Data
Lung and Bronchus Cancer
By Years and Gender**

Year	Males	Females
1994	112	48
1995	121	47
1996	130	49
1997	123	50
1998	121	54
1999	131	55
2000	150	60
2001	155	65
2002	173	72
2003	171	75
2004	172	80
2005	171	83
2006	170	87
2007	168	93
2008	165	120

Preparing Reports

Writing reports for your workplace is not the same as writing an article for a professional journal or preparing a report for an assignment in one of your classes, but the goal is the same. Communication is the goal and it is achieved when you write your report in the style your audience prefers. Often your healthcare administration will let you know how reports are done in your facility, or you could review previous reports that have been given to committees or your administration to use as a guide. Some reports are more formal than others. For example, for a committee meeting you may just provide some data in the form of graphs or tables to share with the members, whereas for a Cancer Conference, where information may be shared with the community, a more formal report will be in order.

Here are some general guidelines to follow:

- Include a title for the report.

- For formal reports or one with many graphs and tables, include a table of contents.

- Include the tables and graphs.

  — Tables and graphs are great tools for presenting data. Tables show summarized and more detailed data and graphs are useful for presenting relationships in visual form. The question of which to use depends on the audience.

  — Take a few minutes before you prepare a report to think about who will be reading or seeing your presentation. Will you be presenting information to your administrator about the need for new equipment in your department; will it be to a team who is deciding whether or not to investigate the need for a new service in your facility; or will it be to a committee evaluating the quality of care provided in your hospital? Determine what you trying to say to this person or group. Determine what details must be included, then decide what types of tables and/or graphs you want to provide.

  — Tables have several advantages over graphs:

    - More information can be presented in a table.

    - Exact values are in tables.

    - Ordinarily less work is involved in creating a table.

  — Graphs, on the other hand, also have advantages:

    - More attention-grabbing than tables.

    - Show trends more clearly.

    - Bring out facts that will stimulate thinking.

- Prepare a narrative report if you are asked to provide one or if the presentation will be more understandable.

  — Tables and graphs are just a part of the decision-making process. Adding narrative discussions to reports help people better understand the data.

  — Narrative description can explain what the values mean.

  — They can include historical information, for instance, what the data has shown over a specific period of time.

  — The narrative can include factors that may influence the data such as seasonal changes in the patient population or reasons for significant increases or decreases in the data.

  — Make sure your data are correct because inaccurate data may lead to inaccurate decisions.

  — Be sure to include the sources of the data.

- Write to the style of your workplace.

  — Be objective. Report all the pertinent information, both positive and negative points.

  — Use bias-free language. Avoid words such as "awesome" or "incredible", etc.

  — Write in an impersonal style. Don't start your sentences with "I compared . . .", but rather, "A comparison showed . . ."

  — Be concise and strive for clarity.

  — Proofread your document; brush-up on your grammatical skills.

Chapter 11 Test

Complete the following exercises.

1. What is one of the simplest types of categorical data where the values fall into unordered categories?

   a. Ordinal
   b. Nominal
   c. Ratio
   d. Interval

2. A graphic display can help healthcare professionals understand data. True or false?

3. What type of numerical data contains only a finite number of results?

   a. Continuous
   b. Discrete

4. In creating a frequency distribution table, which of the following statements is not a basic rule to follow?

   a. Choose classes that cover the smallest and largest values.
   b. Make certain that each item can go into only one class.
   c. As a general rule, use between ten and fifteen classes.
   d. Do not produce gaps between classes.

5. Line graphs can be used to illustrate the relationship between continuous quantities. True or false?

6. When creating histograms, which is a true statement?

   a. Form classes of equal width.
   b. Always form frequency groups that do not overlap.
   c. Establish between five and fifteen frequency groups.
   d. All of the above

(continued on next page)

Chapter 11 Test (continued)

7. Which graph displays vertical bars to depict frequency distributions for continuous data?

   a. Histogram
   b. Line graph
   c. Pie graph
   d. Frequency distribution table

8. Bar graphs are used to display comparisons between nominal data. True or false?

9. What do the wedges or divisions in a pie graph represent?

   a. Frequency groups
   b. Various data
   c. Percentages
   d. Classes

10. Which of the following graphs would be best to use to display the percentages of diagnoses seen at your mental health center?

    a. Frequency polygon
    b. Pie graph
    c. Bar graph
    d. Line graph

11. Which of the following graphs would be best for the cancer registrar to use to display the five-year survival rates of lung cancer patients in the year 20XX to 20XX at your hospital?

    a. Frequency polygon
    b. Bar graph
    c. Line graph
    d. Histogram

12. Which of the following graphs would be best to use to display the number of discharges by medical service for the past year?

    a. Line graph
    b. Bar graph
    c. Histogram
    d. Frequency polygon

Chapter 12
Inferential Statistics in Healthcare

Objectives

At the conclusion of this chapter, you should be able to:

- Define inferential statistics
- Interpret the standard error of the mean and confidence intervals
- Identify and describe the null hypothesis
- Understand the importance of t tests
- Interpret ANOVA
- Understand the significance of chi square

Inferential Statistics

Inferential statistics allow us to generalize from a sample to a population with a certain amount of confidence regarding our findings. Without inferential statistics, it would be very difficult, short of conducting a census, to describe the characteristics of a population. The ability to interpret inferential statistics requires a preexisting understanding of descriptive statistical measures and computations.

Errors in sampling procedures are inevitable; even with random sampling, there is no guarantee that the sample drawn will be representative of the population. For this reason, inferential statistics are limited to certain amounts of confidence.

This chapter discusses the interpretation of common inferential statistical measures, including standard error of the mean, confidence intervals, the null hypothesis, t tests, ANOVA, and chi square.

It is not the intention of this chapter to replace your general statistics course requirement. This chapter merely provides a review of concepts you have learned in that course. An exhaustive explanation of these concepts, including mathematical computation, is beyond the scope of this book.

Standard Error of the Mean and Confidence Intervals

When trying to determine the characteristics of a population, the mean from one sample may not be sufficient because of random sampling error. A more accurate representation could be found by taking many large samples, calculating the mean for each sample, and then finding the standard deviation of all the sample means. This value is called the *standard error of the mean*, abbreviated SE_m, and comes from the standard deviation of many sample means. The graphical representation of all the sample means is a normal distribution when the sample size is reasonably large.

Finding the SE_m in the manner described above can be tedious, and it may not be realistic to find the SE_m of the sample means. For this reason statisticians have found a formula for approximating the SE_m from only one random sample. (A discussion of the theory leading to this formula is not covered in this book.) When the SE_m has been computed, it is generally reported in one of two ways.

1. The data may be displayed in research reports as follows:

$$\bar{X} = 150,\ sd = 10,\ n = 75,\ SE_m = 3$$

Where:

$$\bar{X} = \text{mean}$$

$$sd = \text{standard deviation}$$

$$n = \text{number of observations}$$

$$SE_m = \text{standard error of the mean}$$

Based on the characteristics of the normal curve and treating the SE_m as a margin of error, by adding the SE_m (3) to and subtracting it from the sample mean (150), it can be said with 68.3% confidence that the population mean is somewhere between these two values (147 and 153). This is called a *confidence interval* (abbreviated C.I.).

$$150 - 3 = 147$$

$$150 + 3 = 153$$

Similarly, it can be said with 95.5% confidence that the population mean is between 144 and 156, or two SE_ms.

$$150 - (2 \times 3) = 144$$

$$150 + (2 \times 3) = 156$$

2. The data may be displayed in a research report as follows:

$$\bar{X} = 60, \ sd = 4, \ n = 95, \ SE_m = 1$$

$$68.3\% \text{ C.I.} = 59 \text{ to } 61$$

$$95.5\% \text{ C.I.} = 58 \text{ to } 62$$

$$99.7\% \text{ C.I.} = 57 \text{ to } 63$$

In this example, the confidence intervals have already been computed.

In a normal distribution, confidence intervals are computed by adding one standard error of the mean to and subtracting one from the mean, then adding two standard errors of the mean to and subtracting two from the mean, and so on. The percentages above come from a normal distribution:

68.3% of all scores in a normal distribution fall within + or − 1 standard deviation away from the mean

95.5% of all scores in a normal distribution fall within + or − 2 standard deviations away from the mean

99.7% of all scores in a normal distribution fall within + or − 3 standard deviations away from the mean

A *confidence interval* is the range of scores in which we are estimating the population mean to be. In the example above, the confidence intervals (C.I.) let us know, with a certain amount of confidence, where the mean will lie.

It is important to note that the larger the sample size, the more confidence there is in the mean and the smaller the chance for sampling errors, meaning a smaller SE_m. Further, the more homogenous a population (less variation), the smaller the SE_m. In fact, if a population were all the same (no variation) the SE_m would be zero.

The Null Hypothesis

The *null hypothesis* states that the difference between two population means is zero. This statement is generally made based on two sample means. For example, let's suppose we obtain a sample of the heights of 15-year-old girls at high school A and a second sample of the heights of 15-year-old girls at school B. These are the means:

High school A: $\bar{x} = 5.7$ ft.
High school B: $\bar{x} = 5.6$ ft.

From these results, it would appear that 15-year-old girls at High school A are taller than 15-year-old girls at High school B. However, this may not be true; in fact, the difference may be due to errors in sampling and the mean of the heights of girls at High school A (population mean) may equal the heights of girls at High school B (population mean). This is a statement of a null hypothesis.

The null hypothesis can be expressed as follows:

$H_0: \mu_1 - \mu_2 = 0$

H_0 represents the null hypothesis.

μ_1 represents the population mean for group 1.

μ_2 represents the population mean for group 2.

When conducting research, most researchers are searching for differences in population means and are therefore not looking to confirm the null hypothesis (no differences between the population means). In fact, most research is carried out to reject the null hypothesis. Therefore, researchers may develop an alternative hypothesis to test against the null. The alternative hypothesis can be expressed in one of two ways:

$H_1 = \mu_1 > \mu_2$

H_1 represents the alternative hypothesis.

μ_1 represents the population mean for group 1, hypothesized to be larger than group 2.

μ_2 represents the population mean for group 2, hypothesized to be smaller than group 1.

or

$H_1 = \mu_1 \neq \mu_2$

H_1 represents the alternative hypothesis.

μ_1 represents the population mean for group 1, hypothesized to be different from group 2 without sufficient information to determine which group is larger.

μ_2 represents the population mean for group 2, hypothesized to be different from group 1 without sufficient information to determine which group is larger.

The first alternative hypothesis states that group 1 is larger than group 2; this would be the same as the samples would imply, that 15-year-old girls from High school A are taller than 15-year-old girls from High school B. The second alternative hypothesis states that group 1 and group 2 are different, but there is not enough information to determine which population of girls has the higher mean height.

Because there is always a chance that the null hypothesis is true, testing it will lead to a probability (p) that it is true. The smaller the p value, the more evidence that we should reject the null hypothesis. As a rule of thumb accepted by most statisticians in hypothesis testing, if the probability that the null hypothesis is true is 5% or less, the null hypothesis is rejected.

Rejecting the null hypothesis with this level of confidence is, in effect, describing the relationship between the means as statistically significant. This is generally the manner in which the null hypothesis is discussed in academic journals.

Probabilities of the null hypothesis are expressed as follows:

$p < 5\%$ The probability that the null hypothesis is true is less than 5%

$p < 1\%$ The probability that the null hypothesis is true is less than 1%

$p < 0.1\%$ The probability that the null hypothesis is true is less than 0.1%

Where: p = probability

These different probabilities represent different significance levels; the lower the percentage that the null hypothesis is true, the more significant the finding. Thus, a $p \leq 0.1\%$ is more significant a finding than a $p \leq 5\%$.

Dealing with certain levels of uncertainty creates two types of errors in hypothesis testing: Type I errors and Type II errors. A Type I error occurs when the null hypothesis is rejected, yet it is actually true. A Type II error occurs when the null hypothesis is not rejected, yet it is false. Here are examples of both types of errors:

Type I Error

According to the National Cancer Institute, a woman's chance of being diagnosed with breast cancer from age 50 through age 59 is 2.63%. With this knowledge, going to see a doctor because of a lump on her breast presents a risk that the doctor will diagnose the patient with breast cancer even if she does not have breast cancer. Rejecting the null hypothesis in this instance would be assuming that he will not diagnose her with breast cancer. However, if she is diagnosed with breast cancer, this would be an example of a Type I error. Simply said, the patient could receive a positive test result when, in fact, she does not have breast cancer.

Type II Error

"Suppose a drug company has developed a new drug for a serious disease. Suppose that, in reality, the new drug is effective. If, however, the null hypothesis is not rejected because the drug company selected a level of significance that is too high, the results of the study will have to be described as insignificant and the drug may not receive government approval" (Pyrczak, 2003, 83). This is an example of a Type II error.

When describing the null hypothesis, it is never "accepted." Rather, we say "reject the null hypothesis" or "fail to reject the null hypothesis."

The *t* Test

A *t* test is an example of a test of the null hypothesis to determine if a set of results is statistically significant. As mentioned previously, for the results to be considered statistically significant, the probability that the null hypothesis is true should be 5% or less. The results of a *t* test can be written several ways. Consider the following example.

Example:

Group	$\bar{x}$	standard deviation (sd)	*n*
A	5.3	1.6	10
B	5.5	1.0	10

With this group of data, the results of the *t* test (computed using computer software or a calculator) can be written as follows:

The null hypothesis: There is no difference between the groups.

H_0: $\mu_1 - \mu_2 = 0$ (the difference between the means is zero)

1. Statistically significant ($t = 2.15$, $df = 18$, $p < .05$)

2. Statistically significant at the .05 level ($t = 2.15$, $df = 18$)

3. Reject H_0 at the .05 level ($t = 2.15$, $df = 18$)

Where: t = the value produced by the *t* test

df = degrees of freedom that approximates the sample size. The degrees of freedom are found by taking $n - 1$ for the number of groups. In the sample above, there are two groups, therefore:

$df = (n_1 - 1) + (n_2 - 1)$

$df = (10 - 1) + (10 - 1) = 18$

$df = 18$

Statements 1 through 3 above all reject the null hypothesis and say that there is a statistically significant difference between the sample means of Group A and Group B ($7.9 - 8.1 = -0.2$).

However, the difference between the means may not be statistically significant. Consider the following example.

Example:

Group	$\bar{x}$	standard deviation (sd)	n
A	25	3	8
B	24	3	8

$H_0: \mu_1 - \mu_2 = 0$ (the difference between the means is zero)

1. Not statistically significant ($t = 1.78$, $df = 14$, $p > .05$)

2. H_0 is not rejected at the .05 level ($t = 1.78$, $df = 14$)

These statements do not reject the null hypothesis and say that the difference between the sample means is not statistically significant ($19 - 18 = 1$). The null hypothesis is not rejected because the probability of the null hypothesis actually occurring is greater than 5%; for this reason, it is not statistically significant.

Example:

Group	$\bar{x}$	standard deviation (sd)	n
A	18	2.5	7
B	17	8	7

The null hypothesis: There is no difference between the groups.

$H_0: \mu_1 - \mu_2 = 0$ (the difference between the means is zero)

($t = 2.15$, $df = 12$, $p > .05$)

Exercise 12.1

Given the information in the example above, would you reject the null hypothesis or not? How would you state your findings?

It is important to note that understanding the computation involved in testing the null hypothesis is reserved for an advanced statistics course and is not involved in the daily activities of a healthcare practitioner. How to interpret the results of these tests, however, is important. For this reason, the next two sections on ANOVA and chi square are briefly introduced.

ANOVA

Although t tests are used to test the difference between means, an analysis of variance (ANOVA) test is used to test the differences among two or more means. Sometimes ANOVA is referred to as an F test and, when only two means are tested, will yield a probability that is the same as a t test's probability.

In the following example, the means from four samples are listed. Using ANOVA will demonstrate six differences among the means.

	LOS Group 1: Patients with Private Insurance	LOS Group 2: Patients with Medicare/Medicaid
Males	$\bar{x} = 10$	$\bar{x} = 23$
Females	$\bar{x} = 15$	$\bar{x} = 17$

Males with Private Insurance (Group A): $\bar{x} = 11$

Males with Medicare/Medicaid (Group B): $\bar{x} = 19$

Females with Private Insurance (Group C): $\bar{x} = 17$

Females with Medicare/Medicaid (Group D): $\bar{x} = 20$

Differences yielded by ANOVA:

1. Between A and B

2. Between A and C

3. Between A and D

4. Between B and C

5. Between B and D

6. Between C and D

This is the power of ANOVA, the ability to test many differences among means at once. If the results from an ANOVA are statistically significant (reject the null hypothesis), the researcher's next step is to figure out what differences are significant. However, if the results are not statistically significant (the null hypothesis is not rejected), the work is done.

Chi Square

Chi square, represented by the symbol χ^2 is a test of significance that deals with nominal data and frequencies, specifically data that do not lend themselves to the calculation of standard deviations and means. Using computer software to conduct a chi square test is simple and quickly yields results. Consider the following example.

Example: Employees at a large healthcare facility were randomly asked whether they smoked and whether they had parents who smoked. The results of the 150 employees sampled were:

	Parents who smoke	Parents who do not smoke
Employee smokes	45	25
Employee does not smoke	30	50

These data in this table suggest that those employees with parents who did not smoke were likelier not to smoke (50 vs. 25) than were those employees with parents who smoked (30 vs. 45). From this sample alone, there appears to be a relationship between smoking and having parents who smoke. However, there is a possibility that the null hypothesis is true (the relationship does not exist in this population). This is where a chi square test can help determine whether the relationship is significant. A chi square test using the values above yielded these results:

$$\chi^2 = 10.71, df = 1, p < .01$$

Based on the results, there is a less than 1% chance that the null hypothesis is true. Said another way, the results are statistically significant; there is a relationship between employees who do not smoke having parents who do not smoke.

Notice below that the degrees of freedom are determined differently for chi square. The degrees of freedom are found by taking $(r - 1)$ for the number of categories where $r =$ the number of rows.

$$df = (r - 1)$$
$$df = (2 - 1) = 1$$
$$df = 1$$

Chapter 12 Test

1. Define inferential statistics.

2. Explain the difference between descriptive and inferential statistics.

3. Create a null hypothesis for the following research questions:

   a. What are the differences between emergency room shifts on medication errors?

   b. On a clinical trial of a new drug what will be the effects over a currently used drug?

4. How could you reword these research hypotheses below to null hypotheses?

   a. Smoking during pregnancy increases the risk of a child being born prematurely.

   b. Regular exercise in older adults decreases blood pressure levels.

(continued on next page)

Chapter 12 Test (continued)

5. Based on the results below, how would you describe the relationship between heart attack patients being treated with aspirin and whether or not they lived?

	Male heart attack patients treated with aspirin	Male heart attack patients not treated with aspirin
Males who lived	15	4
Males who did not live	2	8

$$\chi^2 = 8.34, df = 1, p \leq .01$$

6. Using the following information, determine if the differences between the means are significant.

Medical Terminology Class

Group A = Number of word elements remembered by students using flash cards

Group B = Number of word elements remembered by students not using flash cards

Group	$\bar{x}$	standard deviation (sd)	n
A	75	2.0	10
B	50	3.5	10

The null hypothesis: There is no difference between the groups.

$$H_0: \mu_1 - \mu_2 = 0 \text{ (the difference between the means is zero)}$$

$$(t = 2.50, df = 18, p < .05)$$

7. Given the following p values, which would be considered more significant?
   a. $p \leq .3$
   b. $p \leq .02$
   c. $p \leq .25$

8. Given the following null hypothesis, give an example of a Type I error.

   H_0: There is no difference between the number of males or females who go to their primary care physician for an annual exam.

9. Given the following null hypothesis, give an example of a Type II error.

   H_0: There is no difference in the level of understanding of this chapter between students who have previously taken a statistics course and students who have not previously taken a statistics course.

10. Given the following information, determine the 68.3%, 95.5%, and 99.7% confidence intervals.

$$\bar{x} = 4.33, SE_m = 3$$

Chapter 13
Basic Research Principles

Objectives

At the conclusion of this chapter, you should be able to:

- Explain the different types of research
- Describe the difference between quantitative and qualitative research
- Differentiate among research designs: exploratory, historical, descriptive, causal, correlational, evaluation, and experimental
- Describe the steps in the research process
- Explain exploratory and conclusive research design methods
- Describe the various data collection techniques
- Differentiate among the following types of samples: probability and nonprobability; simple random, stratified, cluster, judgment, quota, and convenience
- Define Institutional Review Board (IRB) and understand its role in research
- Define hypothesis
- Define reliability and validity
- Differentiate between primary and secondary research

Basic Research Principles

Research is the search toward the solution of problems. It answers questions that you or others may have and calls attention to theories that may be helpful in predicting future experiences.

Research is done in many fields and may be done in a variety of ways. This chapter covers the basic types of research and the steps in the research process, including data collection techniques and the different types of samples.

Two Types of Research

There are generally two types of research: basic and applied. In **basic research**, the investigator is not concerned with the immediate applicability of his or her results but, rather, tries to look for understanding natural processes. In **applied research**, the investigator has some kind of application in mind and wants to discover information about it that can be used to solve a problem or in some way contribute to society.

Research Methodology

Research methodology is the study of different types of research methods. At a higher and more general level, researchers in research methodology have described two overarching approaches to research: the qualitative approach and the quantitative approach.

Qualitative Research

Qualitative research describes events, persons, and so on without the use of numerical data. An example of qualitative research would be interviews with health information practitioners to determine whether their past healthcare experiences affected their decision to enter the health information field or interviews with mothers of handicapped infants to determine how their lives were affected by the birth of their children. Qualitative research consists of interviews, observations, and written documents that may be used individually or in combination. "The richness of data permits a fuller understanding of what is being studied than could be derived from experimental research methods" (Best and Kahn 1993, 186).

Quantitative Research

Quantitative research uses quantitative methods, or numbers, to describe a study, including some comparisons of the population and statistical analysis to describe the results. Quantitative research consists of observations, experiments, and **surveys**.

Table 13.1 illustrates some characteristics of quantitative and qualitative research.

Table 13.1.   Characteristics of Quantitative and Qualitative Research

Quantitative Research	Qualitative Research
• Uses quantitative methods, including observations, experiments, and surveys	• Describes observations without the use of numerical data, including interviews, observations, and written documents
• Is objective	• Is subjective
• Uses controlled measurements	• Uses uncontrolled observations
• Researcher is removed from the data; is an outside observer	• Researcher is close to the data; has an inside perspective
• Can be generalized and replicated	• Is not generalized and may not be replicable
• Is outcome oriented	• Is process oriented

The Research Process

Although there are as many descriptions of the types of research as there are textbooks and articles about the subject, most agree that the research process involves the following six major steps:

1. Define the problem.
2. Review the literature.
3. Design the research.
4. Collect the data.
5. Analyze the data.
6. Draw conclusions.

Defining the Problem

Problem definition refers to forming a question regarding a topic you would like to study. The most important thing is to be clear about what you want to study. Often an analysis of historical data, or secondary information, has gone into the problem definition.

Historical data analysis simply means looking at the past to see what has been done before; it prevents "reinventing the wheel." In previous research, an investigator may have made recommendations for future studies. In addition, problems may be broken down into subproblems or smaller problems. Figure 13.1 demonstrates an example of a problem and its possible subproblems.

Figure 13.1.   Example of a Research Problem and Its Subproblems

> **Problem/Question:** Should a physician clinic in your community put an organized health information department into operation?
>
> - Subproblem 1. What are the health information services that could be provided?
> - Subproblem 2. What types of employees should be employed in this department?
> - Subproblem 3. What amount of space is needed for the department?
> - Subproblem 4. Where should the health information department be located?
> - Subproblem 5. What equipment does the department need to be operational?
> - Subproblem 6. What would be the total estimated cost of the project?

The definition also may define the scope of the study, that is, who or what will be included in the study. For example, a study that includes hospitals may be defined as including only those hospitals with fewer than 100 beds; a study that involves patients may include only those patients who are age 60 and over; or a study may include females only.

Reviewing the Literature

A **literature review** is an investigation of all the information about a topic. It is important to start any study with a review of literature on the research you want to conduct for three important reasons:

1. to determine whether research has already been done on the question;

2. to determine whether any data sources can be used in the study; and

3. to help make the hypothesis more specific.

There are many sources of previous research. These may include journals, books, position papers, conference presentations, videos, interviews, and online databases, to name just a few.

Designing the Research and Collecting the Data

There are several types of research design, including:

- **Exploratory research** is often undertaken when a problem is not very clearly defined. This type of research allows the researcher to study a problem and gather information. It may generate a hypothesis. Exploratory research is generally informal and relies on literature review and informal discussions with others to find out more about a problem. Although exploratory research may not help answer the problem, it may provide insights into the problem.

- **Historical research** involves an investigation and analysis of past events. This type of research also allows the researcher to apply previous researchers' experiences and conclusions into his or her professional practice.

- **Conclusive research** is performed in order to reach some sort of conclusion or to help in decision making. This type of research may be done using **primary research**, that is, data collected specifically for your study; or **secondary research**, that is, a literature review to see if previous studies can be used to answer your question. Secondary research may also include summaries of past works. There are two types of conclusive research:

    — **Descriptive research**, or statistical research, provides data about the population you are studying, including the frequency that something occurs. These data might include studies on the status of the composition of the HIM work force, employee morale in departments, coding accuracy, or the extent of **electronic health record** (EHR) implementation. The two most common collection techniques for descriptive research are observations and surveys.

    — **Causal research** tries to answer questions about what causes certain things to occur. This type of research is difficult because there may always be an additional cause to consider. Causal research uses experimentation and simulation as its data-collection methods.

- **Correlational research** refers to studies that try to discover a relationship between variables. A variable is anything under study. In correlational research, the strength of the relationship is measured and there may be a positive or a negative relationship between variables. Correlational research only determines if there is a relationship between two or more variables, it does not determine the cause of those relationships. If a strong relationship is found, experimental research can be carried out to determine causality. (See chapter 11 for a more detailed discussion on correlation.) This type of research uses **questionnaires**, observations, and secondary data as its data collection methods. Examples of correlational research might include studying whether there is a relationship between watching violence on television and behavior, whether graduating with a 4.0 average from college affects the type of job a student gets after graduation, or whether there is a relationship between eating eggs and cholesterol levels.

- **Evaluation research** is a process used to determine what has happened during a given activity or in an institution. The purpose of evaluation research is to lead to a better understanding of whether a program is effective, whether a policy is working, or whether something that was agreed upon is the most cost-effective way of doing something. For example, evaluation research may be done each year to determine whether your school's health information program is meeting its goals.

- **Experimental research** entails manipulation of a situation in some way in order to test a hypothesis. In experimental research, certain variables are kept constant and an independent or experimental variable is manipulated. Researchers select both independent and dependent variables. Independent variables are the factors that researchers manipulate directly; dependent variables are the measured variables. Examples of experimental research include studies such as determining whether a certain medication is effective in treating Parkinsonism or studying whether the use of robotic technology in the operating suite is more beneficial to patients than the traditional surgical approach.

Statement of the Hypothesis

In formal research, a **hypothesis** is formed. A hypothesis is a statement of the predicted relationship of what the researcher is studying. It is a proposed solution or explanation the researcher has reached through the literature review. More simply stated, it is the tentative answer to the question being studied.

The statement of the hypothesis is important because it allows the researcher to think about the variables and type of research design to use in the study. The research tests the hypothesis, proving it to be positive or negative (correct or incorrect). The fact that a hypothesis is rejected (that is, proven incorrect) does not necessarily mean that the research is poor but, rather, only that the results are different from what was expected. The formulation of the hypothesis in advance of the data-gathering process is necessary for an unbiased investigation.

There are two forms of the hypothesis:

- The **null hypothesis** states that there is no difference between the population means or proportions being compared or that there is no association between the two variables being compared. For example, in a clinical trial of a new medication, the null hypothesis is: The new medication is no better than the current medication. A detailed discussion of the null hypothesis is given in chapter 12.

- The **alternative hypothesis** is a statement of what the study is set up to establish. For example, in the clinical trial of a new medication, the alternative hypothesis is: The new medication is better than the current medication.

Data Collection Techniques

Data collection includes primary research, or the data obtained from observations, surveys, and interviews. It also includes secondary research, or the literature review or summaries of original studies. Regardless of the data collection method used, the research must be valid and reliable.

- **Validity** is the degree to which scientific observations actually measure or record what they purport to measure. For example, if the researcher is using a written questionnaire to collect data, he or she will pretest it by giving it to someone who may have been included in the subject population in order to determine whether it is well written, clear, and inclusive of everything the researcher is looking for.

- **Reliability** is the repeatability of scientific observations. With reliability, the major question is: Can another researcher reproduce the study using a similar instrument and get similar results? A study may be reliable, but not valid. That is, the study may be able to be replicated and yet not answer the research question.

The type of data collection technique used depends on the type of research the investigator wishes to conduct. If the researcher wants to establish a causal relationship, he or she should conduct one of the experimental studies. However, if the researcher is breaking new ground in a poorly understood area of practice, he or she may want to consider an exploratory study in a qualitative design.

Some examples of data collection methods include:

- *Surveys:* The survey method gathers data from a relatively large number of cases at a particular time. Surveys can include interviews and questionnaire surveys. In either case, the questions should be well-thought out to ensure that they answer the questions of the research study. The questions can be restricted, or closed ended, when the investigator only wants certain answers. For example, "Yes" and "No" answers fall into this category. It is a good idea to provide for unanticipated responses. Providing an "other" category permits respondents to indicate what might be their most important reason, one the questionnaire builder had not anticipated. Open-ended or **unrestricted questions** allow the participant to express a freer response in his or her own words. Open-ended questionnaires can be difficult to tabulate, and although they can be easier to write, it may be better to take additional time to write a closed-form type of questionnaire because it is easier to interpret and tabulate. When standardized questions are used in the interview process, this is referred to as a **structured interview**.

- *Observation:* Instead of asking questions, the investigator observes the participant.

  — In nonparticipant observation, the researcher is a neutral observer who does not interact with the participants.

  — In participant observation, the researcher may participate in the actions being observed but tries to maintain his or her objectivity.

  — Another type of observation is called **ethnography**, or **naturalistic observation**. Using this method of observation, the researcher observes, listens to, and sometimes converses with the subjects in as free and natural an atmosphere as possible. The assumption is that the most important behavior of individuals in groups is a dynamic process of complex interactions and consists of more than one set of facts, statistics, or even discrete incidents. A position of neutrality is important in this type of research.

- *Experimental study:* "This type of data collection technique provides a logical, systematic way to answer the question. If this is done under carefully controlled conditions, what will happen?" (Best and Kahn 1993, 162). There are many types of experimental studies, and a complete discussion would be too lengthy and complex for this introductory section. Experimentation is a sophisticated technique for the collection of data and may not be appropriate for the beginning investigator.

Selection of an Instrument

The **instrument**, also called a tool, is a consistent way to collect data. Many different types of instruments are used in research studies, and whatever type is used should be one that fits the purpose of the research.

Researchers sometimes use instruments that have been published in databases and occasionally publish their own instrument with their research. However, researchers should not develop an instrument until they have established that one does not already exist. If you decide to develop your own instrument, develop the questions carefully and be sure to test them to ensure that you are gathering what you need to answer the question in your research problem. It would be too costly and time-consuming to have to repeat a survey because a question or two had been neglected.

Selection of Samples

Another consideration in data collection is the selection of subjects for the study. For example, a study on health information departments in the United States could try to include every HIM department in the nation, but it would likely prove impractical and could be costly and time-consuming. The next best thing is to use a **sample**. When chosen correctly, samples are considered to be representative of the population.

Generally, there are two types of sampling techniques: probability sampling and non-probability sampling. Probability sampling uses some form of random selection. Probability sampling includes the following three types:

- Simple **random sampling**: This sampling technique involves choosing individuals from the population in such a way that every individual has an equal chance of being selected.

  Statistics books include a table of random numbers that can be used in the selection of random samples. In order to draw a random sample, the researcher should begin by assigning a number to each subject in the population. This number is dependent on the number of subjects in the population. For example, if there are 105 subjects in the population, the first subject would be numbered 001, the second 002 and so on with the final subject being number 105. Similarly, if there are 2,582 subjects in the population, the first subject would be numbered 0001, the second 0002 and the last subject being numbered 2,582. The researcher must begin by selecting subjects at random using the table of random numbers. This can be done by moving across or down the table, as long as the correct number of digits is selected. If the population contains 1,000 subjects, each time the researcher selects a subject, he must select four digits. If he comes across a number not included in the number of subjects (for example, the researcher comes across 8,569, but only has 1,000 subjects), this number is simply discarded and the he moves onto the next number.

  — In **systematic random sampling**, a systematic pattern is used with random sampling. For example, if you were choosing a list of patients discharged during the past month, you might choose the first patient randomly and every fifth patient thereafter. In this sample, choice of the first patient determines the others.

- **Stratified random sampling**: To select a stratified random sample, divide the population into groups of similar individuals, called strata, choose a separate simple random sample (SRS) in each stratum, and then combine the SRSs to form the full sample. For example, you might want to make a selection based on gender, by patients with private insurance, or by separating hospitals by **bed size**.

- **Cluster sampling**: In this technique, the population is selected from groups, or clusters. For example, if the study includes HIM practitioners working in large cities, you first would choose the cities (the cluster) and then randomly choose the HIM practitioners. This is called two-stage cluster sampling.

Almost all qualitative research methods rely on nonprobability sampling. Nonprobability sampling does not involve a random sampling of the population. Nonprobability sampling includes:

- **Judgment sampling**: In judgment sampling, the researcher relies on his or her own judgment to select subjects for a study. For example, in a study on health information departments in acute care hospitals that are using an electronic health record, the researcher might use his or her judgment to select a specific hospital size for the study from among large, small, and medium-sized hospitals that use electronic health records.

- **Quota sampling**: In this type of sampling technique, the researcher first divides the population, as in stratified sampling, and then selects the number of subjects based on a specified proportion. Continuing with the example of health information departments above, if 50 of the 100 hospitals in the state are using an electronic health record and 50 are not, the researcher may choose to base his or her study on 20 of the hospitals because that would be 20 percent of the total population of hospitals in the state.

- **Convenience sampling**: In this sampling technique, selection is based on the availability of subjects. Continuing with the example above, the researcher may decide to use only hospitals within a specific city or within a certain driving distance.

There also are procedures to consider when performing research studies. Federal regulations require that facilities have an **Institutional Review Board** (IRB) that is responsible for reviewing all research projects. IRB is a common term used in organizations, however, an institution may use whatever name it chooses. Some organizations refer to this group as an Independent Ethics Committee or Human Subjects Committees. The purpose of an IRB is to ensure that steps are being taken by the researcher to protect the rights and welfare of anyone participating in the research study. IRBs are responsible for reviewing the research procedures before the study is started and may require periodic reviews during the study. They may approve, revise, or deny requests for research in their facility. Any research on humans must be done carefully to ensure that subjects are not abused in any way. Referring to the earlier example of a study consisting of interviews with mothers of handicapped infants, although there would not be any physical pain to the mothers, questions asked in the study theoretically could cause the mothers emotional pain. The researcher must obtain permission from the IRB before any research study is started and prepare a plan for the research. This means that the researcher must have thought through the research very carefully, prepared any questionnaires, decided how to select a sample and how to collect data in order to prepare the documentation necessary for the IRB, including informed consent forms for the subjects to read and sign. It is necessary to ask any participants to sign a statement indicating that they understand what will be asked of them. Moreover, the researcher must protect the privacy of any research participants. Information about the federal guidelines may be found at the Office for Human Research Protections of the Department of Health and Human Service Web site. Federal regulations must be followed by all IRBs and individuals when conducting research on human subjects. These can be found in the *Code of Federal Regulations* Title 45 Public Welfare Department of Health and Human Services Part 46 Protection of Human Subjects Effective June 23, 2005.

Some facilities may also have a Research Protocol Monitoring Committee that reviews any research before and during the study to ensure that there are no adverse effects on the participants. It may even recommend closure of research that is not meeting safety standards, does not have scientific merit, or is not meeting the goals of the research.

Sample Size

Usually there is a trade-off between the desirability of a large sample and the feasibility of a small one. The ideal **sample size** is one that is large enough to serve as an adequate representation of the population about which the researcher wishes to generalize and small enough to be selected economically in terms of subject availability, expense in both time and money, and complexity of data analysis. Here are tips about sample size:

- The larger the sample, the smaller the magnitude of sampling error.

- Survey studies ordinarily have a larger sample size than experimental studies.

- Questionnaires that are mailed can have a response rate as low as 20 to 30 percent, so a large initial sample is recommended.

- When planning to have subgroups from the study population, begin with a large group to make sure you have enough participants for the subgroups.

- Subject availability and costs are legitimate considerations in determining appropriate sample size.

Analyzing the Data

In this step of the research process, the investigator tries to determine what the data disclose. Most researchers use a variety of techniques to describe the data. Two types of statistical applications are relevant to most studies:

- Descriptive statistics describe the data. Measures of central tendency and measures of variation are included in descriptive statistics. These are discussed in detail in chapter 10.

- Inferential statistics allow the researcher to make inferences about the population characteristics (parameters) from the sample's characteristics. Analysis of variance (ANOVA) and t tests are examples of inferential statistics that are discussed in chapter 12.

Statistics Software Packages

There are many software packages on the market to help researchers analyze their data. A search on the Internet will give you a listing of hundreds of free software packages. These packages can help the researcher produce descriptive statistics along with charts or graphs. One such package is Epi-Info, which is free software from the Centers for Disease Control and Prevention. It includes a program to create questionnaires along with allowing entry of data and analysis and creation of graphs and charts.

Another package used in the pharmaceutical industry is DecisionSite to help researchers predict a medication's chances for success. This software gives researchers the ability to combine lab data with patient demographics in order to help companies decide which drug to develop and market.

SPSS (Statistical Package for Social Sciences) is a statistical package that provides many industries with analytical software. It also is used by a variety of industries for its predictive analytics ability to help them make decisions.

Drawing Conclusions

Any conclusions reached from the study should be related to the hypothesis, or when using the qualitative approach, the problem identified. The results from each hypothesis should be described. Any limitations discovered during data analysis should be reported. For example, the study of health information departments mentioned earlier studied one city. That may be a limiting factor; that is, perhaps different, or at least additional, data should have been collected from other geographical areas. In the presentation of the research findings, new hypotheses may be proposed if the data do not support the original hypothesis. Researchers usually include tables and graphs in this section of the research report to clarify and display the data.

Research always raises new questions about what to study, and these become suggestions for future research. The researcher should always include conclusions as to whether or not the problem is better understood or perhaps even resolved from the research.

Health information researchers provide other HIM professionals with knowledge and methods to answer questions and to decipher problems in the work setting. Researchers should be commended for their hard work because they must be very patient and unhurried. Research requires expertise and practice and is rarely spectacular work. However, it has contributed not only to a better place to practice health information, but also to a better place to live and a greater understanding of the world around us.

Those students who would like to be involved in research and who need to develop skills in research should follow these steps:

1. Take at least one course in statistics and research methodologies.

2. Begin to read research studies in professional journals to see how others have performed their research.

3. Agree to work with a skilled health information researcher on a study to gain experience. You can find this information by contacting the author of a research study that you enjoyed reading. It is highly likely he or she will be performing another research study.

4. Learn how to present data effectively both in written form and verbally.

Statistics is the servant, not the master, of logic; it is a means rather than an end of research. "Unless basic assumptions are valid, unless the right data are carefully gathered, recorded, and tabulated, and unless the analysis and interpretations are logical, statistics can make no contribution to the search for truth" (Best and Kahn 1993, 316).

Chapter 13 Test

Complete the following exercises.

1. Which of the following is considered to be the search toward the solution of the problem?

    a. Fact
    b. Data
    c. Information
    d. Research

2. What are generally the two types of research?

    a. Basic and applied
    b. Scientific and hypothetical
    c. Theory and hypothesis
    d. Quantitative and qualitative

3. The type of research describing events, persons, and so on without the use of numerical data is called:

    a. Quantitative research
    b. Qualitative research
    c. Theoretical research
    d. Hypothetical research

4. The type of research that uses methods or numbers, including comparisons of population and statistical analysis, to describe results is called:

    a. Quantitative research
    b. Qualitative research
    c. Theoretical research
    d. Hypothetical research

5. Which of the following refers to analysis that looks at the past?

    a. Theoretical analysis
    b. Hypothetical analysis
    c. Historical analysis
    d. Concurrent analysis

6. Which type of research tries to answer questions about what causes certain things to occur?

    a. Historical research
    b. Conclusive research
    c. Descriptive research
    d. Causal research

Chapter 13 Test (continued)

7. Which type of research provides data about the population you are studying and is also called statistical research?

   a. Historical research
   b. Conclusive research
   c. Descriptive research
   d. Causal research

8. Which type of research entails manipulation of a situation in some way in order to test a hypothesis?

   a. Correlational research
   b. Evaluation research
   c. Experimental research
   d. Hypothetical research

9. A statement of the predicted relationship of what the researcher is studying is called a(n):

   a. Educated guess
   b. Hypothesis
   c. Theory
   d. Essay

10. The degree to which scientific observations actually measure or record what they purport to measure is referred to as:

    a. Validity
    b. Reliability
    c. Integrity
    d. Theory

11. Which of the following is the repeatability of scientific observations?

    a. Validity
    b. Reliability
    c. Integrity
    d. Theory

12. Which data collection method gathers data from a relatively large number of cases at a particular time?

    a. Observation
    b. Experimental study
    c. Survey
    d. Essay

(continued on next page)

Chapter 13 Test (continued)

13. This type of sample consists of individuals from the population chosen in such a way that every individual has an equal chance of being selected.

    a. Simple random sample
    b. Quota sample
    c. Cluster sample
    d. Judgment sample

14. In which type of sample does the researcher rely on his or her judgment to select the subjects?

    a. Simple random sample
    b. Quota sample
    c. Cluster sample
    d. Judgment sample

15. Statistics that describe the data are referred to as:

    a. Descriptive statistics
    b. Inferential statistics
    c. Measurement statistics
    d. Integral statistics

References

AHIMA e-HIM Work Group. 2003. Practice brief: Electronic document management as a component of the electronic health record. http://library.ahima.org/xpedio/groups/public/documents/ahima/bok1_021594. hcsp?dDocName=bok1_021594.

AHIMA e-HIM Work Group. 2003. Practice brief: E-mail as a provider–Patient electronic communication medium and its impact on the electronic health record. http://library.ahima.org/xpedio/groups/public/ documents/ahima/bok1_021588.hcsp.

AHIMA e-HIM Work Group on Health Information in a Hybrid Environment. 2003. Practice brief: The complete medical record in a hybrid environment. http://library.ahima.org/xpedio/groups/public/documents/ ahima/bok1_022142.hcsp.

AHIMA E-HIM Work Group on Implementing Electronic Signatures. 2003. Practice brief: Implementing electronic signatures. http://library.ahima.org/xpedio/groups/public/documents/ahima/bok1_021585. hcsp?dDocName=bok1_021585.

Ball, C.N., and J. Conner-Linton. 2003. WebChi Square Calculator. http://www.georgetown.edu/faculty/ballc/ webtools/web_chi.html.

Best, J., and J. Kahn. 1993. *Research in Education.* 7th ed. Boston: Allyn and Bacon.

Centers for Disease Control and Prevention. 2005. Nosocomial Infections Surveillance System (NNIS). http:// www.cdc.gov/ncidod/dhqp/nnis.html.

Dinman, S. 1996. A guide to nursing research. *Plastic Surgical Nursing* 16(2).

Dunn, R. 2003. Calculating costs for accounting of disclosures. *Journal of AHIMA* 74(5): 65–66.

Dunn, R. 2002. Turning production data into management tools. *Journal of AHIMA* 73(9) 60–66.

Dunn, R. 1999. *Finance Principles for the Health Information Manager.* Chicago: AHIMA.

Freund, John E., and Gary A. Simon. 1995. *Statistics: A First Course,* 6th ed. New Jersey: Prentice-Hall.

Garner J. 1985. Guideline for Prevention of Surgical Wound Infections. Hospital Infections Program. Centers for Infectious Diseases Center for Disease Control. http://wonder.cdc.gov/wonder/prevguid/p0000420/ p0000420.asp#head004003000000000.

Gauvreau, K., and M. Pagano. 1993. *Principles of Biostatistics.* Belmont, CA: Duxbury Press.

Johns, M., ed. 2007. *Health Information Management Technology: An Applied Approach,* 2nd ed. Chicago: AHIMA.

Johnson, T. and H. Neill. 2001. *Mathematics.* Chicago: Contemporary Books.

Lane, D.M. 2005. *HyperStat Online Textbook.* http://davidmlane.com/hyperstat/.

LaTour, K. and S. Eichenwald Maki, eds. 2006. *Health Information Management: Concepts, Principles, and Practice,* 2nd ed. Chicago: AHIMA.

Lorence, D. 1999. Productivity: How do you measure up? *Journal of AHIMA* 70(5): 35–39.

Malone, S. 1997. Staffing to volume in integrated delivery networks. *Journal of AHIMA* 68(9): 42–48.

Miller, P. J., and F. L. Waterstraat. 2004. Apples to apples: Using autobenchmarking to measure productivity. *Journal of AHIMA* 75(1): 44–49.

Moore, D. 2000. *The Basic Practice of Statistics.* 2nd ed. New York: W.H. Freeman and Company.

Moore, D.S. 2004. *The Basic Practice of Statistics.* 3rd ed. New York: W.H. Freeman and Company.

National Cancer Institute. 2006. Probability of Breast Cancer in American Women. http://www.cancer.gov/cancertopics/factsheet/Detection/probability-breast-cancer.

National Center for Health Statistics. 2003. National Vital Statistics System. http://www.cdc.gov/nchs/nvss.htm.

National Center for Health Statistics. 2005. Deaths/Mortality (U.S.) Final Data for 2005. http://www.cdc.gov/nchs/fastats/deaths.htm.

National Center for Health Statistics. 2008. National Vital Statistics Reports: Deaths, Final Data for 2006. http://www.cdc.gov/nchs/data/nvsr/nvsr57/nvsr57_14.pdf

National Conference of State Legislatures, 2008 Certificate of Need: State Laws and Programs. http://www.ncsl.org/programs/health/cert-need.htm.

National Institutes of Health, Public Health Service. *Statistics and Epidemiology for Cancer Registries.* SEER Program Self-Instructional Manual for Cancer Registrars, Book 7. Washington, DC: U.S. Department of Health and Human Services.

National Program of Cancer Registrars; United States Cancer Statistics. 1999–2004 Cancer Incidence and Mortality Data. http://apps.nccd.cdc.gov/uscs/.

Osborn, C. 2000. *Statistical Applications for Health Information Management.* Gaithersburg, MD: Aspen.

Pronovost, P, D. Angus, T. Dorman, K Robinson, T. Dremsizov, T. Young. 2002. Physician staffing patterns and clinical outcomes in critically ill patients. *JAMA* 288(17): 2151–62.

Pyrczak, F. 2003. *Making Sense of Statistics: A Conceptual Overview.* Los Angeles: Pyrczak Publishing.

Rahal, Lois, RN, BSN, CIC, Infection Control Nurse, Wesley Medical Center, Wichita, KS. Interview December 23, 2008.

Reswick, J, 1994. What constitutes valid research? Qualitative vs. quantitative research. *Journal of Rehabilitation Research and Development.* 31(2).

Rudner, L. and W.D. Schafer. 1999. How to write a scholarly report. *Practical Assessment, Research & Evaluation* 6(13). http://pareonline.net/getvn.asp?v=6&n=13.

Salkind, N. 2004. *Statistics for People Who (Think They) Hate Statistics.* Thousand Oaks, CA: Sage Publications.

U.S. Census Bureau. National and State Population Estimates 2000–2005. http://www.census.gov/popest/states/NST-ann-est2005.html.

U.S. Department of Health and Human Services. Hospital Compare. http://www.hospitalcompare.hhs.gov/Hospital/Search/Welcome.asp?version=default&browser=IE%7C6%7CWinXP&language=English&defaultstatus=0&pagelist=Home.

WebMD. 2009. Types of Anesthesia. http://www.webmd.com/pain-management/tc/anesthesia-types-of-anesthesia

Appendix A
Formulae

Formulae Listed Alphbetically by Name

Adjusted Hospital Autopsy Rate (p. 101) [Chapter 7]

$$\frac{\textit{Total hospital autopsies} \times 100}{\textit{Total number of deaths of hospital patients whose bodies are available for autopsy}}$$

Anesthesia Death Rate (p. 80) [Chapter 6]

$$\frac{\textit{Total deaths caused by anesthetic agents} \times 100}{\textit{Total number of anesthetics administered}}$$

Average Daily Inpatient Census (p. 38) [Chapter 3]

$$\frac{\textit{Total inpatient service days for a period (excluding newborns)}}{\textit{Total number of days in the period}}$$

Average Daily Newborn Census (p. 39) [Chapter 3]

$$\frac{\textit{Total newborn inpatient service days for a period}}{\textit{Total number of days in the period}}$$

Average Length of Stay (p. 62) [Chapter 5]

$$\frac{\textit{Total length of stay (discharge days)}}{\textit{Total discharges (including deaths)}}$$

Average Newborn Length of Stay (p. 63) [Chapter 5]

$$\frac{Total\ newborn\ discharge\ days}{Total\ newborn\ discharges\ (including\ deaths)}$$

Bed Occupancy Ratio (p. 46) [Chapter 4]

$$\frac{Total\ inpatient\ service\ days\ in\ a\ period \times 100}{Total\ bed\ count\ days\ in\ the\ period\ (Bed\ count \times Number\ of\ days\ in\ the\ period)}$$

Bed Turnover Rate, Direct Formula (p. 53) [Chapter 4]

$$\frac{Number\ of\ discharges\ (including\ deaths)\ for\ a\ period}{Average\ bed\ count\ during\ the\ period}$$

Bed Turnover Rate, Indirect Formula (p. 53) [Chapter 4]

$$\frac{Occupancy\ Rate \times Number\ of\ days\ in\ a\ period}{Average\ length\ of\ stay}$$

Cancer Mortality Rate (p. 89) [Chapter 6]

$$\frac{Number\ of\ cancer\ deaths\ during\ a\ period \times 100}{Total\ number\ in\ population\ at\ risk}$$

Case Fatality Rate (p. 73) [Chapter 6]

$$\frac{Number\ of\ people\ who\ die\ of\ a\ disease\ in\ a\ specified\ period \times 100}{Number\ of\ people\ who\ have\ the\ disease}$$

Case-Mix (p. 156) [Chapter 9]

$$\frac{Sum\ of\ the\ weights\ of\ MS\text{-}DRGs\ (Medicare\ severity\ diagnosis\text{-}related\ groups)\ for\ patients\ discharged\ during\ a\ given\ period}{Total\ number\ of\ patients\ discharged}$$

Cesarean-Section Rate (p. 123) [Chapter 8]

$$\frac{Total\ number\ of\ C\text{-}sections\ performed\ in\ a\ period \times 100}{Total\ number\ of\ deliveries\ in\ the\ period\ (including\ C\text{-}sections)}$$

Consultation Rate (p. 125) [Chapter 8]

$$\frac{Total\ number\ of\ patients\ receiving\ a\ consultation \times 100}{Total\ number\ of\ patients\ discharged}$$

Fetal Autopsy Rate (p. 105) [Chapter 7]

$$\frac{Autopsies\ performed\ on\ intermediate\ and\ late\ fetal\ deaths\ for\ a\ period \times 100}{Total\ intermediate\ and\ late\ fetal\ deaths\ for\ the\ same\ period}$$

Fetal Death Rate (p. 88) [Chapter 6]

$$\frac{Total\ number\ of\ intermediate\ and/or\ late\ fetal\ deaths\ for\ a\ period \times 100}{Total\ number\ of\ live\ births\ +\ Intermediate\ and\ late\ fetal\ deaths\ for\ the\ period}$$

Gross Autopsy Rate (p. 96) [Chapter 7]

$$\frac{Total\ autopsies\ on\ inpatient\ deaths\ for\ a\ period \times 100}{Total\ inpatient\ deaths\ for\ the\ period}$$

Gross (Hospital) Death Rate (p. 73) [Chapter 6]

$$\frac{Number\ of\ inpatient\ deaths\ (including\ NB)\ in\ a\ period\ \times 100}{Number\ of\ discharges\ (including\ A\&C\ and\ NB\ deaths)\ in\ the\ same\ period}$$

Infant mortality rate (p. 86) [Chapter 6]

$$\frac{Number\ of\ infant\ deaths\ (neonatal\ and\ postneonatal)\ during\ a\ period \times 1,000}{Number\ of\ live\ births\ during\ the\ period}$$

Infection Rate (p. 117) [Chapter 8]

$$\frac{Total\ number\ of\ infections \times 100}{Total\ number\ of\ discharges\ (including\ deaths)\ for\ the\ period}$$

Labor Productivity (p. 146) [Chapter 9]

$$Completed\ work = Total\ work\ output - Defective\ work$$

$$Labor\ productivity = \frac{Completed\ work}{Hours\ worked\ to\ produce\ total\ work\ output}$$

Maternal Death Rate (p. 82) [Chapter 6]

$$\frac{Number\ of\ direct\ maternal\ deaths\ for\ a\ period \times 100}{Number\ of\ obstetrical\ discharges\ (including\ deaths)\ for\ the\ period}$$

Neonatal Mortality Rate (p. 86) [Chapter 6]

$$\frac{Number\ of\ neonatal\ deaths\ during\ a\ period \times 1,000}{Number\ of\ live\ births\ during\ the\ period}$$

Net Autopsy Rate (p. 98) [Chapter 7]

$$\frac{\textit{Total autopsies on inpatient deaths for a period} \times 100}{\textit{Total inpatient deaths} - \textit{Unautopsied coroners' or medical examiners' cases}}$$

Net Death Rate (p. 76) [Chapter 6]

$$\frac{\textit{Total number of inpatient deaths (including NB) minus deaths} < 48 \textit{ hours for a given period} \times 100}{\textit{Total number of discharges (including NB deaths) minus deaths} < 48 \textit{ hours from the same period}}$$

Newborn Autopsy Rate (p. 104) [Chapter 7]

$$\frac{\textit{Newborn autopsies for a period} \times 100}{\textit{Total newborn deaths for the period}}$$

Newborn Bassinet Occupancy Ratio (p. 51) [Chapter 4]

$$\frac{\textit{Total newborn inpatient service days for a period} \times 100}{\textit{Total newborn bassinet count} \times \textit{Number of days in the period}}$$

Newborn Mortality Rate (p. 85) [Chapter 6]

$$\frac{\textit{Total number of newborn deaths for a period} \times 100}{\textit{Total number of newborn discharges (including deaths) for the period}}$$

Nosocomial Infection Rate (p. 116) [Chapter 8]

$$\frac{\textit{Total number of nosocomial infections for a period} \times 100}{\textit{Total number of discharges, including deaths, for the same period}}$$

Other Rates (p. 128) [Chapter 8]

$$\frac{\textit{Number of times something happened} \times 100}{\textit{Number of times something could have happened}}$$

Payback Period (p. 152) [Chapter 9]

$$\frac{\textit{Total cost of project}}{\textit{Annual incremental cash flow}}$$

Postoperative Death Rate (p. 77) [Chapter 6]

$$\frac{\textit{Total number of deaths (within 10 days after surgery)} \times 100}{\textit{Total number of patients who were operated on for the period}}$$

Postoperative Infection Rate (p. 120) [Chapter 8]

$$\frac{\textit{Total number of infections in clean surgical cases for a period} \times 100}{\textit{Number of surgical operations for the period}}$$

Rate (p. 18) [Chapter 2]

$$Rate = \frac{Part}{Base}, \text{ or } R = \frac{P}{B}$$

Return on Investment (p. 152) [Chapter 9]

$$\frac{\textit{Average annual incremental cash flow}}{\textit{Total cost of the project}}$$

Staffing Level (p. 146) [Chapter 9]

$$\frac{\textit{Patient encounters}}{\textit{Productivity}} = \textit{Number of FTEs needed}$$

Standard Deviation (p. 183) [Chapter 10]

$$SD = \sqrt{\frac{\sum (X - \bar{X})^2}{(N-1)}}$$

Unit Labor Costs (p. 136) [Chapter 9]

$$\frac{\textit{Total (sum) medical transcriptionist annual compensation}}{\textit{Total (sum) medical transcriptionist annual productivity}}$$

Variance (p. 180) [Chapter 10]

$$s^2 = \frac{(X_1 - \bar{X})^2 + (X_2 - \bar{X})^2 + (X_3 - \bar{X})^2 \textit{ and so on}}{N-1}$$

Vital Statistics Maternal Mortality Rate (p. 82) [Chapter 6]

$$\frac{\textit{Number of deaths attributed to maternal conditions during a period} \times 100,000}{\textit{Number of births during the period}}$$

Formulae Listed by Chapter in Which They Appear

Chapter 2

Rate (p. 18)

Chapter 3

Average Daily Inpatient Census (p. 38)
Average Daily Newborn Census (p. 39)

Chapter 4

Bed Occupancy Ratio (p. 46)
Bed Turnover Rate, Direct Formula (p. 53)
Bed Turnover Rate, Indirect Formula (p. 53)
Newborn Bassinet Occupancy Ratio (p. 51)

Chapter 5

Average Length of Stay (p. 62)
Average Newborn Length of Stay (p. 63)

Chapter 6

Anesthesia Death Rate (p. 80)
Cancer Mortality Rate (p. 89)
Case Fatality Rate (p. 73)
Fetal Death Rate (p. 88)
Gross (Hospital) Death Rate (p. 73)
Infant Mortality Rate (p. 86)
Maternal Death Rate (p. 82)
Neonatal Mortality Rate (p. 86)
Net Death Rate (p. 76)
Newborn Mortality Rate (p. 85)
Postoperative Death Rate (p. 77)
Vital Statistics Maternal Mortality Rate (p. 82)

Chapter 7

Adjusted Hospital Autopsy Rate (p. 101)
Gross Autopsy Rate (p. 96)
Fetal Autopsy Rate (p. 105)
Net Autopsy Rate (p. 98)
Newborn Autopsy Rate (p. 104)

Chapter 8

Chapter 9

Chapter 10

Appendix B
Glossary of Healthcare Services and Statistical Terms

Accuracy: A characteristic of data that are free from significant error, up-to-date, and representative of relevant facts

Adjusted hospital autopsy rate: The proportion of hospital autopsies performed following the deaths of patients whose bodies are available for autopsy

Admission date: In the home health prospective payment system, the date of first service; in the acute care prospective payment system, the year, month, and day of inpatient admission, beginning with a hospital's formal acceptance of a patient who is to receive healthcare services while receiving room, board, and continuous nursing services

Aggregate data: Data extracted from individual health records and combined to form de-identified information about groups of patients that can be compared and analyzed

Alternative hypothesis: A hypothesis that states that there is an association between independent and dependent variables

Ambulatory care: Preventive or corrective healthcare services provided on a nonresident basis in a provider's office, clinic setting, or hospital outpatient setting

Ancillary service visit: The appearance of an outpatient in a unit of a hospital or outpatient facility to receive services, tests, or procedures that ordinarily are not counted as encounters for healthcare services

Ancillary services: Tests and procedures ordered by a physician to provide information for use in patient diagnosis or treatment

Anesthesia death rate: The ratio of deaths caused by anesthetic agents to the number of anesthetics administered during a specified period of time

Applied research: A type of research that focuses on the use of scientific theories to improve actual practice as in medical research applied to the treatment of patients

Arithmetic mean length of stay (AMLOS):   The average length of stay for all patients

Autopsy: The postmortem examination of the organs and tissues of a body to determine the cause of death or pathological conditions

Autopsy rate: The proportion or percentage of deaths in a healthcare organization that are followed by the performance of an autopsy

Available for hospital autopsy: A situation in which the required conditions have been met to allow an autopsy to be performed on a hospital patient who has died

Average: The value obtained by dividing the sum of a set of numbers by the number of values

Average daily census: The mean number of hospital inpatients present in the hospital each day for a given period of time

Average duration of hospitalization: *See* **Average length of stay**

Average length of stay (ALOS):   The mean length of stay for hospital inpatients discharged during a given period of time

Bar chart: A graphic technique used to display frequency distributions of nominal or ordinal data that fall into categories; also called bar graph

Bar graph: *See* **Bar chart**

Basic research: A type of research that focuses on the development and refinement of theories

Bed capacity: The number of beds that a facility has been designed and constructed to house

Bed complement: *See* **Bed count**

Bed count: The number of inpatient beds set up and staffed for use on a given day; also called bed complement

Bed count day: A unit of measure that denotes the presence of one inpatient bed (either occupied or vacant) set up and staffed for use in one 24-hour period

Bed occupancy ratio: The proportion of beds occupied, defined as the ratio of inpatient service days to bed count days during a specified period of time

Bed size: The total number of inpatient beds for which a facility is equipped and staffed to provide patient care services

Bed turnover rate: The average number of times a bed changes occupants during a given period of time

Boarder: An individual such as a parent, caregiver, or other family member who receives lodging at a healthcare facility but is not a patient

Boarder baby: A newborn who remains in the nursery following discharge because the mother is still hospitalized, or a premature infant who no longer needs intensive care but remains for observation

Budget: A plan that converts the organization's goals and objectives into targets for revenue and spending

Calculation of inpatient service days: The measurement of the services received by all inpatients in one 24-hour period

Calculation of transfers: A medical care unit that shows transfers on and off the unit as subdivisions of patients admitted to and discharged from the unit

Cancer mortality rate: The proportion of patients that die from cancer

Case fatality rate: The total number of deaths due to a specific illness during a given time period divided by the total number of cases during the same period

Case-mix index: The average relative weight of all cases treated at a given facility or by a given physician, which reflects the resource intensity or clinical severity of a specific group in relation to the other groups in the classification system

Categorical data: Four types of data (nominal, ordinal, interval, and ratio) that represent values or observations that can be sorted into a category; also called scales of measurement

Causal research: A type of conclusive research that tries to answer questions about what causes certain things to occur.

Cause-specific death rate: The total number of deaths due to a specific illness during a given time period divided by the estimated population for the same time period

Census: The number of inpatients present in a healthcare facility at any given time

Census day: *See* **Inpatient service day**

Census statistics: Statistics that examine the number of patients being treated at specific times, the lengths of their stay, and the number of times a bed changes occupants

Census survey: A survey that collects data from all the members of a population

Centers for Disease Control and Prevention (CDC):   A group of federal agencies that oversees health promotion and disease control and prevention activities in the United States

Centers for Medicare and Medicaid Services (CMS):   The division of the Department of Health and Human Services that is responsible for developing healthcare policy in the United States and for administering the Medicare program and the federal portion of the Medicaid program; called the Health Care Financing Administration (HCFA) prior to 2001

Certificate of need: A state-directed program that requires healthcare facilities to submit detailed plans and justifications for the purchase of new equipment, new buildings, or new service offerings that cost in excess of a certain amount

Cesarean-section rate: The ratio of all Cesarean sections to the total number of deliveries, including Cesarean sections, during a specified period of time

Chronic: Of long duration

Clean surgical case: A surgical case in which no infection existed prior to surgery

Clinic outpatient: A patient who is admitted to a clinical service of a clinic or hospital for diagnosis or treatment on an ambulatory basis

Clinical research: A specialized area of research that primarily investigates the efficacy of preventive, diagnostic, and therapeutic procedures; also called medical research

Cluster sampling: The process of selecting subjects for a sample from each cluster within a population (for example, a family, school, or community)

Community-acquired infection: An infectious disease contracted as the result of exposure before or after a patient's period of hospitalization

Complete master census: A total census for a facility showing the names and locations of patients present in the hospital at a particular point in time

Complication: A medical condition that arises during an inpatient hospitalization (for example, a postoperative wound infection)

Conclusive research: A type of research performed in order to come to some sort of conclusion or help in decision making; includes descriptive research and causal research

Concomitant: Accessory; taking place at the same time

Consultation: The response by one healthcare professional to another healthcare professional's request to provide recommendations and/or opinions regarding the care of a particular patient/resident

Consultation rate: The total number of hospital inpatients receiving consultations for a given period divided by the total number of discharges and deaths for the same period

Continuous data: Data that represent measurable quantities but are not restricted to certain specified values

Control group: A comparison study group whose members do not undergo the treatment under study

Convenience sampling: A sampling technique where the selection of units from the population is based on easy availability and/or accessibility

Coroner: A public officer whose principal duty is to inquire via an inquest into the cause of any death that there is reason to suppose is not due to natural causes

Coroner's case: A death that appears to be suspicious and requires action from the coroner to determine the cause of death

Correlational research: A design of research that determines the existence and degree of relationships among factors

Cost–benefit analysis: A process that uses quantitative techniques to evaluate and measure the benefit of providing products or services compared to the cost of providing them

Crude birth rate: The number of live births divided by the population at risk

Crude death rate: The total number of deaths in a given population for a given period of time divided by the estimated population for the same period of time

Daily census: The number of inpatients present at the census-taking time each day, plus any inpatients who were both admitted after the previous census-taking time and discharged before the next census-taking time

Daily inpatient census: The number of inpatients present at census-taking time each day, plus any inpatients who were both admitted and discharged after the census-taking time the previous day

Data: The dates, numbers, images, symbols, letters, and words that represent basic facts and observations about people, processes, measurements, and conditions

Data accuracy: The extent to which data are free of identifiable errors

Data collection: The process by which data are gathered

Date of encounter (outpatient and physician services):   The year, month, and day of a visit, or other healthcare encounter

Date of procedure (inpatient):   The year, month, and day of each significant procedure

Date of service (DOS):   The date a test, procedure, and/or service was rendered

Days of stay: *See* **Length of stay**

Dead on arrival (DOA):   The condition of a patient who arrives at a healthcare facility with no signs of life and who was pronounced dead by a physician

Death rate: The proportion of inpatient hospitalizations that end in death

Decile: The tenth equal part of a distribution

Decimal: Numbered or proceeding by tens; based on the number 10; expressed in or utilizing a decimal system, especially with a decimal point

Delivery: The process of delivering a liveborn infant or dead fetus (and placenta) by manual, instrumental, or surgical means

Denominator: The part of a fraction below the line signifying division that functions as the divisor of the numerator and, in fractions with 1 as the numerator, indicates into how many parts the unit is divided

Dependent variable: A measurable variable in a research study that depends on an independent variable

Descriptive research: A type of conclusive research that determines and reports the current status of topics and subjects

Descriptive statistics: Statistics that describe populations

Discharge date (inpatient):   The year, month, and day that an inpatient was formally released from the hospital and room, board, and continuous nursing services were terminated

Discharge days: *See* **Length of stay** and **Total length of stay**

Discharge diagnosis list: A complete set of discharge diagnoses applicable to a single patient episode, such as an inpatient hospitalization

Discharge transfer: The transfer of an inpatient to another healthcare institution at the time of discharge

Discrete data: Data that represent separate and distinct values or observations; that is, data that contain only finite numbers and have only specified values

Disposition: For outpatients, the healthcare practitioner's description of the patient's status at discharge (no follow-up planned; follow-up planned or scheduled; referred elsewhere; expired); for inpatients, a core health data element that identifies the circumstances under which the patient left the hospital (discharged alive; discharged to home or self-care; discharged and transferred to another short-term general hospital for inpatient care;

discharged and transferred to a skilled nursing facility; discharged and transferred to an intermediate care facility; discharged and transferred to another type of institution for inpatient care or referred for outpatient services to another institution; discharged and transferred to home under care of organized home health services organization; discharged and transferred to home under care of a home intravenous therapy provider; left against medical advice or discontinued care; expired; status not stated)

Duration of inpatient hospitalization: *See* **Length of stay**

Early fetal death: The death of a product of human conception that is fewer than twenty weeks of gestation and 500 grams or less in weight before its complete expulsion or extraction from the mother

Electronic health record (EHR):   A computerized record of health information and associated processes; also called computer-based patient record

Electronic medical record (EMR):   A form of computer-based health record in which information is stored in whole files instead of by individual data elements

Electronic signature: Any representation of a signature in digital form, including an image of a handwritten signature; also, the authentication of a computer entry in a health record made by the individual making the entry

Emergency patient: A patient who is admitted to the emergency services department of a hospital for the diagnosis and treatment of a condition that requires immediate medical, dental, or allied health services in order to sustain life or to prevent critical consequences

Encounter: The direct personal contact between a patient and a physician or other person authorized by state licensure law and, if applicable, by medical staff bylaws to order or furnish healthcare services for the diagnosis or treatment of the patient

Episode of care: A period of relatively continuous medical care performed by healthcare professionals in relation to a particular clinical problem or situation

Ethnography: A method of observational research that investigates culture in naturalistic settings using both qualitative and quantitative approaches

Evaluation research: A design of research that examines the effectiveness of policies, programs, or organizations

Exacerbation: To make more violent, bitter, or severe

Experimental research: A research design used to establish cause and effect; also, a controlled investigation in which subjects are assigned randomly to groups that experience carefully controlled interventions that are manipulated by the experimenter according to a strict protocol; also called experimental study

Exploratory research: A research design used because a problem has not been clearly defined or its scope is unclear

Fetal autopsy rate: The number of autopsies performed on intermediate and late fetal deaths for a given time period divided by the total number of intermediate and late fetal deaths for the same time period

Fetal death: The death of a product of human conception before its complete expulsion or extraction from the mother regardless of the duration of the pregnancy; also called stillborn

Fetal death rate: A proportion that compares the number of intermediate and/or late fetal deaths to the total number of live births and intermediate or late fetal deaths during the same period of time

Fiscal year: Any consecutive twelve-month period an organization uses as its accounting period

Fraction: One or more parts of a whole

Frequency distribution: A table or graph that displays the number of times (frequency) a particular observation occurs

Frequency distribution table: A table consisting of a set of classes or categories along with the numerical counts that correspond to nominal and ordinal data

Frequency polygon: A type of line graph that represents a frequency distribution

Full-time equivalent employees (FTEs): The total number of workers, including part-time, in an area as the equivalent of full-time positions

Gender: The biological sex of the patient as recorded at the start of care

Graph: A graphic tool used to show numerical data in a pictorial representation

Gross autopsy rate: The number of inpatient autopsies conducted during a given time period divided by the total number of inpatient deaths for the same time period

Gross death rate: The number of inpatient deaths that occurred during a given time period divided by the total number of inpatient discharges, including deaths, for the same time period

Histogram: A graphic technique used to display the frequency distribution of continuous data (interval or ratio data) as either numbers or percentages in a series of bars

Historical research: A research design used to investigate past events

Home health (HH): An umbrella term that refers to the medical and nonmedical services provided to patients and their families in their places of residence; also called home care

Home health agency (HHA): A program or organization that provides a blend of home-based medical and social services to homebound patients and their families for the purpose of promoting, maintaining, or restoring health or of minimizing the effects of illness, injury, or disability

Hospice: An interdisciplinary program of palliative care and supportive services that addresses the physical, spiritual, social, and economic needs of terminally ill patients and their families

Hospice care: The medical care provided to persons with life expectancies of six months or less who elect to forgo standard treatment of their illness and to receive only palliative care

Hospital: A healthcare entity that has an organized medical staff and permanent facilities that include inpatient beds and continuous medical/nursing services; and that provides diagnostic and therapeutic services for patients, as well as overnight accommodations and nutritional services

Hospital ambulatory care: All hospital-directed preventive, therapeutic, and rehabilitative services provided by physicians and their surrogates to patients who are not hospital inpatients

Hospital autopsy: A postmortem (after death) examination performed on the body of a person who has at some time been a hospital patient by a hospital pathologist or a physician of the medical staff who has been delegated the responsibility

Hospital autopsy rate: The total number of autopsies performed by a hospital pathologist for a given time period divided by the number of deaths of hospital patients (inpatients and outpatients) whose bodies were available for autopsy for the same time period

Hospital death rate: The number of inpatient deaths for a given period of time divided by the total number of live discharges and deaths for the same time period

Hospital inpatient: A patient who is provided with room, board, and continuous general nursing services in an area of an acute care facility where patients generally stay at least overnight

Hospital inpatient autopsy: A postmortem (after-death) examination performed on the body of a patient who died during an inpatient hospitalization by a hospital pathologist or a physician of the medical staff who has been delegated the responsibility

Hospital inpatient beds: Accommodations with supporting services (such as food, laundry, and housekeeping) for hospital inpatients, excluding those for the newborn nursery, but including incubators and bassinets in nurseries for premature or sick newborn infants

Hospital live birth: In an inpatient facility, the complete expulsion or extraction of a product of human conception from the mother, regardless of the duration of pregnancy, which, after such expulsion or extraction, breathes or shows any other evidence of life, such as beating of the heart, pulsation of the umbilical cord, or definite movement of voluntary muscles

Hospital newborn bassinet: Accommodations including incubators and isolettes in the newborn nursery with supporting services (such as food, laundry, and housekeeping) for hospital newborn inpatients

Hospital newborn inpatient: A patient born in the hospital at the beginning of the current inpatient hospitalization

Hospital outpatient: A hospital patient who receives services in one or more of a hospital's facilities when he or she is not currently an inpatient or a home care patient

Hospital outpatient care unit: An organized unit of a hospital that provides facilities and medical services exclusively or primarily to patients who are generally ambulatory and who do not currently require or are not currently receiving services as an inpatient of the hospital

Hospital-acquired infection: *See* **Nosocomial infection**

Hospitalization: The period during an individual's life when he or she is a patient in a single hospital without interruption except by possible intervening leaves of absence

Hybrid health record: A combination of paper and electronic records

Hypothesis: A statement that describes a research question in measurable terms

Iatrogenic: Induced inadvertently by a physician or surgeon or by medical treatment or diagnostic procedures

Incidence rate: A computation that compares the number of new cases of a specific disease for a given time period to the population at risk for the disease during the same time disease (or a disease that developed during pregnancy, labor, or the puerperium) that was not due to obstetric causes, although the physiologic effects of pregnancy were partially responsible for the death

Induced termination of pregnancy: The purposeful interruption of an intrauterine pregnancy that was not intended to produce a liveborn infant and that did not result in a live birth

Infant death: The death of a liveborn infant at any time from the moment of birth to the end of the first year of life (364 days, twenty-three hours, fifty-nine minutes from the moment of birth)

Infant mortality rate: The number of deaths of individuals under one year of age during a given time period divided by the number of live births reported for the same time period

Infection rate: The ratio of all infections to the number of discharges, including deaths

Inferential statistics: Statistics that are used to make inferences from a smaller group of data to a large one

Information: Data that have been deliberately selected, processed, and organized to be useful

Inpatient: *See* **Hospital inpatient**

Inpatient admission: An acute care facility's formal acceptance of a patient who is to be provided with room, board, and continuous nursing service in an area of the facility where patients generally stay at least overnight

Inpatient bed count: *See* **Bed count**

Inpatient bed occupancy rate: The total number of inpatient service days for a given time period divided by the total number of inpatient bed count days for the same time period; also called percentage of occupancy

Inpatient census: *See* **Census**

Inpatient days of stay: *See* **Length of stay**

Inpatient discharge: The termination of hospitalization through the formal release of an inpatient from a hospital; *see also* **Discharge**

Inpatient service day: A unit of measure equivalent to the services received by one inpatient during one 24-hour period

Institutional death rate: *See* **Net death rate**

Institutional Review Board (IRB):   An administrative body that provides oversight for the research studies conducted within a healthcare institution

Instrument: A standardized and uniform way to collect data

Intermediate fetal death: The death of a product of human conception before its complete expulsion or extraction from the mother that is twenty completed weeks of gestation (but less than twenty-eight weeks) and weighs 501 to 1,000 grams

Internal validity: An attribute of a study's design that contributes to the accuracy of its findings

Interval data: A type of data that represents observations that can be measured on an evenly distributed scale beginning at a point other than true zero

Interview guide: A list of written questions to be asked during an interview

Intrahospital transfer: A change in medical care unit, medical staff unit, or responsible physician during hospitalization

Intrarater reliability: A measure of a research instrument's reliability in which the same person repeating the test will get reasonably similar findings

Judgment sampling: A sampling technique where the researcher relies on his or her own judgment to select the subjects

Knowledge: The information, understanding, and experience that give individuals the power to make informed decisions

Late fetal death: The death of a product of human conception that is twenty-eight weeks or more of gestation and weighs 1,001 grams or more before its complete expulsion or extraction from the mother

Leave of absence: The authorized absence of an inpatient from a hospital or other facility for a specified period of time occurring after admission and prior to discharge

Leave of absence day: A day occurring after the admission and prior to the discharge of a hospital inpatient when the patient is not present at the census-taking hour because he or she is on leave of absence from the healthcare facility

Length of stay (LOS):   The total number of patient days for an inpatient episode, calculated by subtracting the date of admission from the date of discharge

Line graph: A graphic technique used to illustrate the relationship between continuous measurements; consists of a line drawn to connect a series of points on an arithmetic scale and is often used to display time trends

Literature review: A systematic investigation of all the knowledge available about a topic from sources such as books, journal articles, theses, and dissertations

Low-birth-weight neonate: Any newborn baby, regardless of gestational age, whose weight at birth is less than 2,500 grams

Managed care: A generic term for reimbursement and delivery systems that integrate the financing and provision of healthcare services by means of entering contractual agreements with selected providers to furnish comprehensive healthcare services and developing explicit criteria for the selection of healthcare providers, formal programs of ongoing quality improvement and utilization review, and significant financial incentives for members to use providers associated with the plan

Managed care organization (MCO):   A type of healthcare organization that delivers medical care and manages all aspects of the care or the payment for care by limiting providers of care, discounting payment to providers of care, and/or limiting access to care

Maternal death: The death of any woman, from any cause, related to or aggravated by pregnancy or its management (regardless of duration or site of pregnancy), but not from accidental or incidental causes

Maternal death rate: For a hospital, the total number of maternal deaths directly related to pregnancy for a given time period divided by the total number of obstetrical discharges for the same time period; for a community, the total number of deaths attributed to maternal conditions during a given time period in a specific geographic area divided by the total number of live births for the same time period in the same area

Mean: A measure of central tendency that is determined by calculating the arithmetic average of the observations in a frequency distribution

Measure: A term referring to the quantifiable data about a function or process

Measurement: The systematic process of data collection, repeated over time or at a single point in time

Measures of central tendency: The typical or average numbers that are descriptive of the entire collection of data for a specific population

Median: A measure of central tendency that shows the midpoint of a frequency distribution when the observations have been arranged in order from lowest to highest

Medical examiner: *See* **Coroner**

Medical services: The activities relating to medical care performed by physicians, nurses, and other healthcare professional and technical personnel under the direction of a physician

Method: A way of performing an action or task; also, a strategy used by a researcher to collect, analyze, and present data

Mode: A measure of central tendency that consists of the most frequent observation in a frequency distribution

Morbidity: A term referring to the state of being diseased (including illness, injury, or deviation from normal health); the number of sick persons or cases of disease in relationship to a specific population

Morgue: The place where the bodies of persons who have died are kept until identified and claimed by relatives or are released for burial

Mortality: A term referring to the incidence of death in a specific population; also, the loss of subjects during the course of a clinical research study, or attrition

Mortality rate: A rate that measures the risk of death for the cause under study in a defined population during a given time period

Multivariate: In reference to research studies, a term meaning that many variables were involved

Naturalistic observation: A type of nonparticipant observation in which researchers observe certain behaviors and events as they occur naturally

Necropsy: *See* **Autopsy**

Neonatal death: The death of a liveborn infant within the first twenty-seven days, twenty-three hours, and fifty-nine minutes following the moment of birth

Neonatal mortality rate: The number of deaths of infants under twenty-eight days of age during a given time period divided by the total number of births for the same time period

Neonatal period: The period of an infant's life from the hour of birth through the first twenty-seven days, twenty-three hours, and fifty-nine minutes of life

Net autopsy rate: The ratio of inpatient autopsies compared to inpatient deaths calculated by dividing the total number of inpatient autopsies performed by the hospital pathologist for a given time period by the total number of inpatient deaths minus unautopsied coroners' or medical examiners' cases for the same time period

Net death rate: The total number of inpatient deaths minus the number of deaths that occurred less than forty-eight hours after admission for a given time period divided by the total number of inpatient discharges minus the number of deaths that occurred less than forty-eight hours after admission for the same time period

Newborn (NB):   An inpatient who was born in a hospital at the beginning of the current inpatient hospitalization

Newborn autopsy rate: The number of autopsies performed on newborns who died during a given time period divided by the total number of newborns who died during the same time period

Newborn bassinet count: The number of available hospital newborn bassinets, both occupied and vacant, on any given day

Newborn bassinet count day: A unit of measure that denotes the presence of one newborn bassinet, either occupied or vacant, set up and staffed for use in one 24-hour period

Newborn mortality rate: The number of newborns who died divided by the total number of newborns, both alive and dead

Nominal data: A type of data that represents values or observations that can be labeled or named and where the values fall into unordered categories; also called dichotomous data

Normal distribution: A continuous frequency distribution characterized by a bell-shaped curve; that is, the mean, median, and mode are equal and most of the measurements are near the center of the frequency

Nosocomial infection: An infection acquired by a patient while receiving care or services in a healthcare organization; also called hospital-acquired infection

Nosocomial infection rate: The number of hospital-acquired infections for a given time period divided by the total number of inpatient discharges for the same time period

Null hypothesis: A hypothesis that states there is no association between the independent and dependent variables in a research study

Numerator: The part of a fraction that is above the line and signifies the number of parts of the denominator taken

Numerical data: Data that include discrete data and continuous data

Nursing facility: A comprehensive term for long-term care facilities that provide nursing care and related services on a 24-hour basis for residents requiring medical, nursing, or rehabilitative care

Observation patient: A patient who presents with a medical condition with a significant degree of instability and disability and who needs to be monitored, evaluated, and assessed to determine whether he or she should be admitted for inpatient care or discharged for care in another setting

Occasion of service: A specified, identifiable service that involves the care of a patient but is not an encounter (for example, a lab test ordered during an encounter)

Occupancy percent/ratio: *See* **Bed occupancy ratio**

Operation: *See* **Surgical operation**

Ordinal data: A type of data that represents values or observations that can be ranked or ordered

Outlier: An extreme statistical value that falls outside the normal range

Outpatient: A patient who receives ambulatory care services in a hospital-based clinic or department

Patient: A living or deceased individual who is receiving or has received healthcare services

Patient care unit (PCU):   An organizational entity of a healthcare facility organized both physically and functionally to provide care

Patient day: *See* **Inpatient service day**

Payback period: A financial method used to evaluate the value of a capital expenditure by calculating the time frame that must pass before inflow of cash from a project equals or exceeds outflow of cash

Percentage: A value computed on the basis of the whole divided into 100 parts

Percent/percentage of occupancy: *See* **Inpatient bed occupancy rate**

Perinatal death: An all-inclusive term that refers to both stillborn infants and neonatal deaths

Pictogram: A graphic technique in which pictures are used in the display of data

Pie chart: A graphic technique in which the proportions of a category are displayed as portions of a circle (like pieces of a pie)

Pie graph: *See* **Pie chart**

Population: The universe of data under investigation from which a sample is taken

Postmortem examination: *See* **Autopsy**

Postneonatal death: The death of a liveborn infant from twenty-eight days to the end of the first year of life (three hundred sixty-four days, twenty-three hours, and fifty-nine minutes from the moment of birth)

Postneonatal mortality rate: The number of deaths of persons aged twenty-eight days up to, but not including, one year during a given time period divided by the number of live births for the same time period

Postoperative death rate: The ratio of deaths within ten days after surgery to the total number of operations performed during a specified period of time

Postoperative infection rate: The number of infections that occur in clean surgical cases for a given time period divided by the total number of operations within the same time period

Postpartum: Occurring after childbirth

Postterm neonate: Any neonate whose birth occurs from the beginning of the first day (two hundred ninety-fifth day) of the forty-third week following onset of the last menstrual period

Preexisting condition: Any injury, disease, or physical condition occurring prior to an arbitrary date

Prepartum: Occurring prior to childbirth

Preterm infant: An infant with a birth weight between 1,000 and 2,499 grams and/or a gestation between twenty-eight and thirty-seven completed weeks

Preterm neonate: Any neonate whose birth occurs through the end of the last day of the thirty-eighth week (two hundred sixty-sixth day) following onset of the last menstrual period

Primary data source: Record developed by healthcare professionals in the process of providing patient care

Primary research: Data collected specifically for a study

Procedure: *See* **Surgical procedure**

Productivity: A unit of performance defined by management in quantitative standards

Profiling: A measurement of the quality, utilization, and cost of medical resources provided by physicians that is made by employers, third-party payers, government entities, and other purchasers of healthcare

Proportion: The relation of one part to another or to the whole with respect to magnitude, quantity, or degree

Puerperal: The period immediately following childbirth

Qualitative research: A philosophy of research that assumes that multiple contextual truths exist and bias is always present; also called qualitative research; also called naturalism

Quantitative research: A philosophy of research that assumes that there is a single truth across time and place, and that researchers are able to adopt a neutral, unbiased stance and establish causation; also called positivism

Quartile: The fourth equal part of a distribution

Questionnaire: A type of survey in which the members of the population are questioned through the use of electronic or paper forms

Quota sampling: A sampling technique where the population is first segmented into mutually exclusive subgroups, just as in stratified sampling, and then judgment is used to select the subjects or units from each segment based on a specified proportion

Quotient: The number resulting from the division of one number by another

Random sampling: An unbiased selection of subjects that includes methods such as simple random sampling, stratified random sampling, systematic sampling, and cluster sampling

Randomization: The assignment of subjects to experimental or control groups based on chance

Range: Distance or extent between possible extremes

Ranked data: A type of ordinal data where the observations are first arranged from highest to lowest according to magnitude and then assigned numbers that correspond to each observation's place in the sequence

Rate: A measure used to compare an event over time; a comparison of the number of times an event did happen (numerator) with the number of times an event could have happened (denominator)

Ratio: A calculation found by dividing one quantity by another; also, a general term that can include a number of specific measures such as proportion, percentage, and rate

Ratio data: Data that may be displayed by units of equal size and placed on a scale starting with zero and thus can be manipulated mathematically (for example, 0, 5, 10, 15, 20)

Recap: Abbreviation of *recapitulation*

Recapitulation: A concise summary of data

Recurrence: To occur again after an interval

Relevance: How applicable information is to some matter

Reliability: A measure of consistency of data items based on their reproducibility and an estimation of their error of measurement

Research: Investigation or experimentation aimed at the discovery and interpretation of facts, revision of accepted theories or laws in the light of new facts, or practical application of such new or revised theories or laws; the collecting of information about a particular subject

Research data: Data used for the purpose of answering a proposed question or testing a hypothesis

Return on investment (ROI): The financial analysis of the extent of value a major purchase will provide

Rounding: The process of approximating a number

Run chart: A type of graph that shows data points collected over time and identifies emerging trends or patterns

Sample: A set of units selected for study that represents a population

Sample size: The number of subjects needed in a study to represent a population

Sample size calculation: The qualitative and quantitative procedures to determine an appropriate sample size

Sample survey: A type of survey that collects data from representative members of a population

Scales of measurement: *See* **Categorical data**

Scatter diagram: A graph that visually displays the linear relationships among factors

Secondary data source: Data derived from the primary patient record, such as an index or database

Secondary record: A record derived from the primary record and containing selected data elements

Secondary research: Data collected from a literature review

Skewness: The horizontal stretching of a frequency distribution to one side or the other so that one tail is longer than the other

Standard deviation: A measure of variability that describes the deviation from the mean of a frequency distribution in the original units of measurement; the square root of the variance

Statistics: A branch of mathematics concerned with collecting, organizing, summarizing, and analyzing data

Stillbirth: The birth of a fetus, regardless of gestational age, that shows no evidence of life (such as heartbeats or respirations) after complete expulsion or extraction from the mother during childbirth

Stratified random sampling: The process of selecting the same percentages of subjects for a study sample as they exist in the subgroups (strata) of the population

Structured interview: An interview format that uses a set of standardized questions that are asked of all applicants

Surgical death rate: *See* **Postoperative death rate**

Surgical operation: One or more surgical procedures performed at one time for one patient via a common approach or for a common purpose

Surgical procedure: Any single, separate, systematic process upon or within the body that can be complete in itself; is normally performed by a physician, dentist, or other licensed practitioner; can be performed with or without instruments; and is performed to restore disunited or deficient parts, remove diseased or injured tissues, extract foreign matter, assist in obstetrical delivery, or aid in diagnosis

Survey: A type of research instrument with which the members of the population being studied are asked questions and respond orally

Systematic random sampling: The process of selecting a sample of subjects for a study by drawing every *n*th unit on a list

Table: An organized arrangement of data, usually in columns and rows

Term neonate: Any neonate whose birth occurs from the beginning of the first day of the thirty-ninth week (two hundred sixty-seventh day) through the end of the last day of the forty-second week (two hundred ninety-fourth day), following onset of the last menstrual period

Total bed count days: The sum of inpatient bed count days for each of the days during a specified period of time.

Total discharge days: *See* **Total length of stay**

Total inpatient service days: The sum of all inpatient service days for each of the days during a specified period of time

Total length of stay: The sum of the days of stay of any group of inpatients discharged during a specific period of time; also called discharge days

Transfer: The movement of a patient from one treatment service or location to another; *see also* **Intrahospital transfer**

Unit labor cost: Cost determined by dividing the total annual compensation by total annual productivity

Unrestricted question: A type of question that allows free-form responses; also called open-ended question

Utilization management: A program that evaluates the healthcare facility's efficiency in providing necessary care to patients in the most effective manner

Validity: The extent to which data correspond to the actual state of affairs or that an instrument measures what it purports to measure; also, a term referring to a test's ability to accurately and consistently measure what it purports to measure.

Variability: The difference between each score and every other score in a frequency distribution.

Variable: A characteristic or property that may take on different values.

Variance: A disagreement between two parts; the square of the standard deviation

Variance analysis: An assessment of a department's financial transactions to identify differences between the budget amount and the actual amount of a line item

Visit: A single encounter with a healthcare professional that includes all the services supplied during the encounter

Vital statistics: Data related to births, deaths, marriages, and fetal deaths

Well newborn: A newborn born at term, under sterile conditions, with no diseases, conditions, disorders, syndromes, injuries, malformations, or defects diagnosed, and no operations other than routine circumcision performed

Whole number: Any of the set of nonnegative integers

Appendix C
Answers to Odd-Numbered Chapter Exercises

Chapter 2

Exercise 2.1

1. $\dfrac{40}{80} = \dfrac{4}{8} = \dfrac{1}{2}$

2. $\dfrac{3}{9} = \dfrac{1}{3}$

3. $\dfrac{75}{150} = \dfrac{1}{2}$

4. $\dfrac{6}{36} = \dfrac{1}{6}$

5. $\dfrac{20}{100} = \dfrac{2}{10} = \dfrac{1}{5}$

Exercise 2.3

1. $48 = 50$
2. $356 = 360$
3. $311 = 310$
4. $5,896 = 5,900$
5. $3,258 = 3,260$
6. $9,631 = 9,630$
7. $232,563 = 232,560$
8. $2,634 = 2,630$
9. $48,605 = 48,610$
10. $8,563 = 8,560$
11. $651 = 700$
12. $123 = 100$
13. $8,307 = 8,300$
14. $7,534 = 7,500$
15. $5,781 = 5,800$
16. $18.3 = 18$
17. $32.5 = 33$
18. $23.1 = 23$
19. $152.6 = 153$
20. $99.4 = 99$
21. $15.89 = 15.9$
22. $18.58 = 18.6$
23. $32.62 = 32.6$
24. $99.98 = 100.0$
25. $124.07 = 124.1$

Exercise 2.5

1. $14:28 = 7:14 = 1:2$
2. $3:12 = 1:4$
3. $5:10 = 1:2$
4. $7:49 = 1:7$
5. $1:16 = 1:16$

Chapter 3

Exercise 3.1

1. Yes. The counts could have differed. Any number of admissions, discharges, or transfers could have occurred between 12 midnight and 1 a.m. on either day.

2. No. The total hospital census would be inconsistent. Every PCU in the hospital should follow the same administrative procedures.

3. No. The patient cannot be in two places at the same time. If both units are counting heads only once a day at midnight, the patient is counted as being present in unit A only. However, the patient is indicated in unit B's census as a transfer.

Exercise 3.3

Inpatient daily census will be the same as the figure representing an inpatient service day for any one day. The census represents the number of patients present in the hospital at any one time; it does not refer to the census-taking hour nor does it reflect the patients admitted and discharged the same day.

Exercise 3.5

1. c. Both a and b

2. c. Total inpatient service days

3. b. Consistent

4. a. Counted where he or she is

5. a. Inpatient service day

6. d. 59

7. a. The number of inpatients present in a healthcare facility at any given time

   b. The number of inpatients present at the census-taking time each day, plus any inpatients who were both admitted after the previous census-taking time and discharged before the next census-taking time

   c. A unit of measure equivalent to the services received by one inpatient during one 24-hour period

   d. The sum of all inpatient service days for each of the days during a specified period of time

Exercise 3.7

Day	12:01 a.m. census A/C	Nb	adm A/C	b	trf in	total A/C	Nb	dis A/C	dis Nb	trf out	11:59 p.m. census A/C	Nb	a/d	serv days A/C	Nb
6/1	250	18	20	4	2	**272**	**22**	25	3	2	**245**	**19**	1	246	19
6/2	**245**	**19**	22	6	1	**268**	**25**	24	5	1	**243**	**20**	0	243	20
6/3	**243**	**20**	24	5	0	**267**	**25**	23	4	0	**244**	**21**	3	247	21
6/4	**244**	**21**	22	3	1	**267**	**24**	22	3	1	**244**	**21**	1	245	21
6/5	**244**	**21**	25	4	2	**271**	**25**	25	3	2	**244**	**22**	2	246	22

Exercise 3.9

	Monthly Compilation of Inpatient Census and Inpatient Service Days May 20XX														
Day	12:01 a.m. Census A/C	NB	Adm A/C	bir	trf in	Total A/C	NB	Disch A/C	NB	Trf out	11:59 p.m. Census A/C	NB	A/D	Serv days A/C	NB
1	162	2	22	1	10	194	3	19	0	10	165	3	1	166	3
2	165	3	29	0	8	**202**	**3**	23	1	8	**171**	**2**	0	**171**	**2**
3	**171**	**2**	14	2	3	**188**	**4**	24	0	3	**161**	**4**	1	**162**	**4**
4	**161**	**4**	24	0	5	**190**	**4**	25	0	5	**160**	**4**	0	**160**	**4**
5	**160**	**4**	11	1	6	**177**	**5**	25	2	6	**146**	**3**	0	**146**	**3**
6	**146**	**3**	20	0	1	**167**	**3**	16	0	1	**150**	**3**	0	**150**	**3**
7	**150**	**3**	29	0	10	**189**	**3**	17	0	10	**162**	**3**	0	**162**	**3**
8	**162**	**3**	24	2	13	**199**	**5**	20	0	13	**166**	**5**	3	**169**	**5**
9	**166**	**5**	23	1	7	**196**	**6**	22	1	7	**167**	**5**	1	**168**	**5**
10	**167**	**5**	19	0	10	**196**	**5**	17	0	10	**169**	**5**	0	**169**	**5**
11	**169**	**5**	11	0	5	**185**	**5**	22	3	5	**158**	**2**	1	**159**	**2**
12	**158**	**2**	16	0	6	**180**	**2**	24	0	6	**150**	**2**	0	**150**	**2**
13	**150**	**2**	18	1	5	**173**	**3**	25	0	5	**143**	**3**	0	**143**	**3**
14	**143**	**3**	29	0	5	**177**	**3**	19	0	5	**153**	**3**	0	**153**	**3**
15	**153**	**3**	28	0	8	**189**	**3**	22	2	8	**159**	**1**	1	**160**	**1**
16	**159**	**1**	26	3	6	**191**	**4**	19	0	6	**166**	**4**	0	**166**	**4**
17	**166**	**4**	26	0	7	**199**	**4**	19	2	7	**173**	**2**	0	**173**	**2**
18	**173**	**2**	18	0	10	**201**	**2**	25	0	10	**166**	**2**	0	**166**	**2**
19	**166**	**2**	12	0	6	**184**	**2**	33	0	6	**145**	**2**	0	**145**	**2**
20	**145**	**2**	22	1	8	**175**	**3**	16	3	8	**151**	**0**	1	**152**	**0**
21	**151**	**0**	26	0	3	**180**	**0**	17	0	3	**160**	**0**	1	**161**	**0**
22	**160**	**0**	32	2	11	**203**	**2**	25	0	11	**167**	**2**	1	**168**	**5**

Monthly Compilation of Inpatient Census and Inpatient Service Days May 20XX

	12:01 a.m. Census		Adm		trf	Total		Disch		Trf	11:59 p.m. Census			Serv days	
Day	A/C	NB	A/C	bir	in	A/C	NB	A/C	NB	out	A/C	NB	A/D	A/C	NB
23	**167**	**2**	29	2	14	**210**	**4**	27	0	14	**169**	**4**	0	**169**	**4**
24	**169**	**4**	22	0	10	**201**	**4**	21	2	10	**170**	**2**	0	**170**	**2**
25	**170**	**2**	20	3	13	**203**	**5**	34	0	13	**156**	**5**	0	**156**	**5**
26	**156**	**5**	14	0	6	**176**	**5**	37	1	6	**133**	**4**	1	**134**	**4**
27	**133**	**4**	23	0	5	**161**	**4**	16	0	5	**140**	**4**	0	**140**	**4**
28	**140**	**4**	26	2	4	**170**	**6**	18	2	4	**148**	**4**	0	**148**	**4**
29	**148**	**4**	17	0	6	**171**	**4**	22	1	6	**143**	**3**	1	**144**	**3**
30	**143**	**3**	19	0	7	**169**	**3**	21	1	7	**141**	**2**	0	**141**	**2**
31	**141**	**2**	21	1	12	**174**	**3**	16	0	12	**146**	**3**	1	**147**	**3**
Tot			670	22				686	21				14	4868	91

Recap of Monthly Data for Adults and Children: May 20XX (Enter numbers from Worksheet #1)

12:01 a.m. Census A/C		162
Adm A/C	+	**670**
Trf in	+	**230**
Total A/C	=	**1,062**
Disch A/C	–	**686**
Trf out	–	**230**
11:59 p.m. Census A/C	=	146

Recap of Monthly Data for Newborns:

12:01 a.m. Census NB		2
Bir	+	**22**
Total NB	=	**24**
Disch NB	–	**21**
11:59 p.m. Census NB	=	3

Serv days A/C (total inpatient service days excluding newborns): **4,868**

Serv days NB (total newborn service days): **91**

Total inpatient service days: 4,959

Chapter 4

Exercise 4.1
1. No.

Exercise 4.3

Children's Hospital
April, 20XX

Unit	Bed Count	Inpatient Service Days	Percentage of Occupancy
Pediatric Medicine	55	1,450	$\dfrac{(1,450 \times 100)}{(55 \times 30)} = 87.9\%$
Pediatric Surgery	40	1,059	$\dfrac{(1,059 \times 100)}{(40 \times 30)} = 88.3\%$
Respiratory	25	642	$\dfrac{(642 \times 100)}{(25 \times 30)} = 85.6\%$
Hematology/Oncology	38	1,122	$\dfrac{(1,122 \times 100)}{(38 \times 30)} = 98.4\%$
Pediatric ICU	12	275	$\dfrac{(275 \times 100)}{(12 \times 30)} = 76.4\%$
Pediatric Cardiac ICU	10	261	$\dfrac{(261 \times 100)}{(10 \times 30)} = 87.0\%$
Neonatal ICU	20	456	$\dfrac{(456 \times 100)}{(20 \times 30)} = 76.0\%$

$$\textbf{TOTAL} = \frac{(5,265 \times 100)}{(200 \times 30)} = \frac{526,500}{6,000} = 87.75 = 87.8\%$$

Exercise 4.5

Community Hospital
December, 20XX

PCU	Inpatient Service Days	Bed Count	Percentage of Occupancy
Med/Surg	1,876	70	$\dfrac{(1,876\times100)}{(70\times31)}=\dfrac{187,600}{2,170}=86.45=86.5\%$
ICU	300	10	$\dfrac{(300\times100)}{(10\times31)}=\dfrac{30,000}{310}=96.77=96.8\%$
CCU	240	8	$\dfrac{(240\times100)}{(8\times31)}=\dfrac{24,000}{248}=96.77=96.8\%$
Rehabilitation	300	12	$\dfrac{(300\times100)}{(12\times31)}=\dfrac{30,000}{372}=80.6\%$
Burn	75	5	$\dfrac{(75\times100)}{(5\times31)}=\dfrac{7,500}{155}=48.38=48.4\%$
Psychiatry	200	15	$\dfrac{(200\times100)}{(15\times31)}=\dfrac{20,000}{465}=43.0\%$
Pediatric	870	30	$\dfrac{(870\times100)}{(30\times31)}=\dfrac{87,000}{930}=93.5\%$
Total	3,861	150	$\dfrac{(3,861\times100)}{(150\times31)}=\dfrac{386,100}{4,650}=83.0\%$
Nursery	280	10	$\dfrac{(280\times100)}{(910\times31)}=\dfrac{28,000}{310}=90.3\%$

Exercise 4.7

Turnover rate (direct formula): $\dfrac{6,500}{200}=32.5$

Turnover rate (indirect formula): $\dfrac{(0.8\times365)}{9}=\dfrac{292}{9}=32.4$

Chapter 5

Exercise 5.1

1.

Admitted	Discharged	Length of Stay
5/3	5/4	**1**
7/2	7/12	**10**
2/14	2/28	**14**
3/25	4/15	**21**
8/27	9/10	**14**

Exercise 5.3

1.

Time Admitted	Time Seen by Physician	Time between Checking in at Reception and Being Seen by Physician
8:00 a.m.	8:17 a.m.	**17 minutes**
1:22 p.m.	2:05 p.m.	**43 minutes**
10:30 a.m.	11:43 a.m.	**73 minutes**

Exercise 5.5

1. $\dfrac{825}{158} = 5.2$ days

2. True, however, this is an instance when the median might be a better choice than the average. There are only four patients in this category and one patient has an LOS quite a bit longer than the others, while another patient has an LOS much less than the others.

3.

University Hospital
May, 20XX

Clinical Units	Discharges	Discharge Days	ALOS
Surgery	1,720	8,627	$\dfrac{8,627}{1,720} = 5.0$
Medicine	1,594	7,852	$\dfrac{7,852}{1,594} = 4.9$
Neurology	988	4,285	$\dfrac{4,285}{988} = 4.3$
Oncology	878	18,588	$\dfrac{18,588}{878} = 21.2$
Obstetrics/Gynecology	588	1,479	$\dfrac{1,479}{588} = 2.5$
Ophthalmology	385	1,154	$\dfrac{1,154}{385} = 3.0$
Orthopedics	651	9,321	$\dfrac{9,321}{651} = 14.3$
Pediatrics	358	2,841	$\dfrac{2,841}{358} = 7.9$
Psychiatry/Human Behavior	156	4,697	$\dfrac{4,697}{156} = 30.1$
Rehabilitation	321	8,057	$\dfrac{8,057}{321} = 25.1$
Urology	89	183	$\dfrac{183}{89} = 2.1$
Total	7,728	66,539	$\dfrac{66,539}{7,728} = 8.6$

Exercise 5.7

1.

Admitted	Discharged	LOS
1/12	1/31	**19**
7/4	7/30	**26**
12/31/2007	2/1/2009	**397**
11/24	11/24	**1**
6/19/2007	1/4/2009	**565**

2. $19 + 26 + 397 + 1 + 565 = 1,008$

3. $\dfrac{92,725}{15,987} = 5.8$ days

4. $\dfrac{11,062}{3,421} = 3.2$ days

5. $\dfrac{51,201}{11,644} = 4.4$ days

6. $\dfrac{32,103}{4,852} = 6.6$ days

7. $\dfrac{10,438}{2,912} = 3.4$ days

8.

Community Hospital
Medicare Discharge Statistics
July, 20XX

Unit	Medicare Discharges	Medicare Discharge Days	ALOS
Medicine	325	2,375	$\dfrac{2,375}{325} = 7.3$
Surgery	175	2,103	$\dfrac{2,103}{175} = 12.0$
Rehabilitation	298	4,261	$\dfrac{4,261}{298} = 14.3$
Skilled Nursing	305	6,588	$\dfrac{6,588}{305} = 21.6$

Chapter 6

Exercise 6.1

$$\frac{Gross\ Death\ Rate\ (9+1)\times100}{540+62} = \frac{1000}{602} = 1.66\%$$

Exercise 6.3

Net Death Rate:

$$\frac{\begin{array}{c}((5\ A\&C\ deaths+2\ NB\ deaths)-\\ (1\ A\&C\ death\ less\ than\ 48\ hours+1\ NB\ death\ less\ than\ 48\ hours)\times100)\end{array}}{\begin{array}{c}(307\ A\&C\ discharges+5\ A\&C\ deaths)+(62\ NB\ discharges+2\ NB\ deaths)\\ -(1\ A\&C\ death\ less\ than\ 48\ hours+1\ NB\ death\ less\ than\ 48\ hours)\end{array}} = \frac{(7-2)\times100}{(312+64-2)} = \frac{500}{374} = 1.34\%$$

Exercise 6.5

Community Hospital
January–March 20XX
Number of Surgery Patients and Deaths, by Surgeon

Physician Number	No. of Surgery Patients	No. of deaths within 10 days after surgery	Postoperative Death Rate
Dr. 102	180	4	$\frac{(4\times100)}{180} = 2.22\%$
Dr. 237	120	2	$\frac{(2\times100)}{120} = 1.67\%$
Dr. 391	60	1	$\frac{(1\times100)}{60} = 1.67\%$
Dr. 518	65	1	$\frac{(1\times100)}{65} = 1.54\%$
Dr. 637	98	5	$\frac{(5\times100)}{98} = 5.10\%$
Dr. 802	32	3	$\frac{(3\times100)}{32} = 9.38\%$
Dr. 900	64	1	$\frac{(1\times100)}{64} = 1.56\%$

Exercise 6.7

Community Hospital
July–December 20XX
Selected MS-DRGs–Postoperative Deaths
Number of Surgery Patients and Deaths
Surgery Service

MS-DRG	MS-DRG Title	No. of Surgery Patients	No. of deaths within 10 days after surgery	Postoperative Death Rate
338	Appendectomy w complicated principal diag w MCC	8	1	$\dfrac{(1 \times 100)}{8} = 12.50\%$
327	Stomach, esophageal & duodenal proc w CC	67	2	$\dfrac{(2 \times 100)}{67} = 2.99\%$
005	Liver transplant w MCC or intestinal transplant	17	6	$\dfrac{(6 \times 100)}{17} = 35.29\%$
139	Salivary gland procedures	5	1	$\dfrac{(1 \times 100)}{5} = 20.00\%$
405	Pancreas, liver & shunt procedures w MCC	54	3	$\dfrac{(3 \times 100)}{54} = 5.56\%$
625	Thyroid, parathyroid & thyroglossal procedures w MCC	195	2	$\dfrac{(2 \times 100)}{195} = 1.03\%$
736	Uterine & adnexa proc for ovarian or adnexal malignancy w MCC	132	5	$\dfrac{(5 \times 100)}{132} = 3.79\%$
217	Cardiac valve & oth maj cardiothoracic proc w card cath w CC	201	3	$\dfrac{(3 \times 100)}{201} = 1.49\%$
239	Amputation for circ sys disorders exc upper limb & toe w MCC	8	3	$\dfrac{(3 \times 100)}{8} = 37.50\%$
469	Major joint replacement or reattachment of lower extremity w MCC	132	4	$\dfrac{(4 \times 100)}{132} = 3.03\%$
	Totals	819	30	$\dfrac{(30 \times 100)}{819} = 3.66\%$

Exercise 6.9

General anesthesia death rate:

$$\frac{(2 \times 100)}{663} = 0.30\%$$

Regional anesthesia death rate:

$$\frac{(1 \times 100)}{530} = 0.19\%$$

Local anesthesia death rate:

$$\frac{(1 \times 100)}{133} = 0.75\%$$

Exercise 6.11

$$\frac{(2 \times 100)}{134} = 1.49\%$$

Exercise 6.13

$$\frac{(1 \times 100)}{380} = 0.26\%$$

Exercise 6.15

$$\frac{((2+4) \times 100)}{29+2+4} = \frac{600}{35} = 17.14\%$$

Exercise 6.17

Community Hospital
Cancer Registry Annual Report
Selected Cancer Deaths Reported
20XX

Type of Cancer	No. of Discharges	No. of Deaths	Death Rate
Prostate	23	6	$\dfrac{(6 \times 100)}{23} = 26.09\%$
Breast	56	4	$\dfrac{(4 \times 100)}{56} = 7.14\%$
Lung and Bronchus	28	9	$\dfrac{(9 \times 100)}{28} = 32.14\%$
Colon Rectum	39	2	$\dfrac{(2 \times 100)}{39} = 5.13\%$
Uterus	36	5	$\dfrac{(5 \times 100)}{36} = 13.89\%$
Urinary Bladder	15	2	$\dfrac{(2 \times 100)}{15} = 13.33\%$
Non-Hodgkin's Lymphoma	21	6	$\dfrac{(6 \times 100)}{21} = 28.57\%$
Melanoma of the Skin	23	5	$\dfrac{(5 \times 100)}{23} = 21.74\%$
Kidney and Renal Pelvis	15	3	$\dfrac{(3 \times 100)}{15} = 20.00\%$
Ovary	12	5	$\dfrac{(5 \times 100)}{12} = 41.67\%$
Total	**268**	**47**	$\dfrac{(47 \times 100)}{268} = 17.54\%$

Chapter 7

Exercise 7.1
False, the calculation is

$$\frac{(6 \times 100)}{24} = 25.00\%$$

Exercise 7.3
Gross death rate:
$$\frac{(288 \times 100)}{16,523} = 1.74\%$$

Gross autopsy rate:
$$\frac{(185 \times 100)}{288} = 64.24\%$$

Net autopsy rate:
$$\frac{(185 \times 100)}{(288 - 20)} = \frac{18,500}{268} = 69.03\%$$

Exercise 7.5
Gross death rate:
$$\frac{((345 + 3) \times 100)}{(12,924 + 4,332)} = \frac{34,800}{17,256} = 2.02\%$$

Gross autopsy rate:
$$\frac{(159 \times 100)}{(345 + 3)} = \frac{15,900}{348} = 45.69\%$$

Net autopsy rate:
$$\frac{(159 \times 100)}{((345 + 3) - 6)} = \frac{15,900}{342} = 46.49\%$$

Adjusted hospital autopsy rate:
$$\frac{(159 \text{ inpatient autopsies} + 14 \text{ ESD and OPD autopsies}) \times 100}{((345 \text{ A/C deaths} + 3 \text{ NB deaths} + 15 \text{ ESD and OPD deaths}) - 6 \text{ coroner's cases})} = \frac{17,300}{357} = 48.46\%$$

Exercise 7.7
Adjusted hospital autopsy rate:

$$\frac{((8 \text{ inpatient autopsies} + 1 \text{ SNF death} + 1 \text{ ESD death} + 1 \text{ OPD death} + 1 \text{ HHCD death}) \times 100)}{(23 \text{ inpatient deaths} + 1 \text{ SNF death} + 1 \text{ ESD death} + 1 \text{ OPD death} + 1 \text{ HHCD death}) - 1 \text{ coroner's case})} = \frac{1,200}{26} = 46.15\%$$

Exercise 7.9
Newborn autopsy rate:

$$\frac{(1\times100)}{2}=50.00\%$$

Exercise 7.11
Newborn death rate:

$$\frac{(3\ newborn\ deaths\times100)}{620}=0.48\%$$

Fetal death rate:

$$\frac{((4\ intermediate\ fetal\ deaths+2\ late\ fetal\ deaths)\times100)}{(622\ births+4\ intermediate\ fetal\ deaths+2\ late\ fetal\ deaths)}=\frac{600}{628}=0.96\%$$

Newborn autopsy rate:

$$\frac{(1\ newborn\ autopsy\times100)}{3\ newborn\ deaths}=33.33\%$$

Fetal autopsy rate:

$$\frac{((1\ intermediate\ fetal\ death\ autopsy+1\ late\ fetal\ death\ autopsy)\times100)}{(4\ intermediate\ fetal\ deaths+2\ late\ fetal\ deaths)}=\frac{200}{6}=33.33\%$$

Chapter 8

Exercise 8.1
Nosocomial infection rate for adults and children:

$$\frac{(13\times100)}{1,784}=0.73\%$$

Nosocomial infection rate for newborns:

$$\frac{(3\times100)}{123}=2.44\%$$

Total nosocomial infection rate for the hospital:

$$\frac{((13+3)\times100)}{(1,784+123)}=\frac{1,500}{1,907}=0.84\%$$

Gross death rate for this annual period:

$$\frac{((12+1)\times100)}{(1,784+123)}=\frac{1,300}{1,907}=0.68\%$$

Exercise 8.3

Postoperative infection rate:

$$\frac{(12 \times 100)}{2,059} = 0.58\%$$

Postoperative death rate:

$$\frac{(10 \times 100)}{2,053} = 0.49\%$$

Exercise 8.5

$$\frac{(78 \times 100)}{394} = 19.80\%$$

Exercise 8.7

**Community Hospital
Semiannual Statistics
January–June, 20XX**

Service	Discharges	No. of Patients Receiving Consultations	Consultation Rate
Medicine	2,880	864	$\dfrac{(864 \times 100)}{2,880} = 30.00\%$
Surgery	2,160	701	$\dfrac{(701 \times 100)}{2,160} = 32.45\%$
Obstetrics	685	26	$\dfrac{(26 \times 100)}{685} = 3.80\%$
Psychiatric	142	6	$\dfrac{(6 \times 100)}{142} = 4.23\%$
Rehabilitation	156	12	$\dfrac{(12 \times 100)}{156} = 7.69\%$
Pediatrics	251	42	$\dfrac{(42 \times 100)}{251} = 16.73\%$
Newborn	672	2	$\dfrac{(2 \times 100)}{672} = 0.30\%$
Totals	**6,946**	**1,653**	$\dfrac{(1,653 \times 100)}{6,946} = 23.80\%$

Exercise 8.9

University Hospital
Surgery Service
Semiannual Statistics
January–June 20XX

Month	Discharges	No. of Patients Readmitted Within 30 Days of the Previous Discharge	Readmission Rate
January	562	27	$\frac{(27 \times 100)}{562} = 4.80\%$
February	654	32	$\frac{(32 \times 100)}{654} = 4.89\%$
March	678	38	$\frac{(38 \times 100)}{678} = 5.60\%$
April	649	21	$\frac{(21 \times 100)}{649} = 3.24\%$
May	658	25	$\frac{(25 \times 100)}{658} = 3.80\%$
June	667	34	$\frac{(34 \times 100)}{667} = 5.10\%$
Totals	**3,868**	**177**	$\frac{(177 \times 100)}{3,868} = 4.58\%$

Exercise 8.11

**Community Hospital
Semiannual Statistics
July–December 20XX**

Month	No. of Discharges	No. of Accounts Turned over to a Collection Agency	Rate of Accounts Turned over to a Collection Agency
July	302	25	$\dfrac{(25 \times 100)}{302} = 8.28\%$
August	326	30	$\dfrac{(30 \times 100)}{326} = 9.20\%$
September	342	32	$\dfrac{(32 \times 100)}{342} = 9.36\%$
October	318	15	$\dfrac{(15 \times 100)}{318} = 4.72\%$
November	352	24	$\dfrac{(24 \times 100)}{352} = 6.82\%$
December	312	19	$\dfrac{(19 \times 100)}{312} = 6.09\%$
Totals	**1,952**	**145**	$\dfrac{(145 \times 100)}{1,952} = 7.43\%$

Exercise 8.13

Medicine service rate compared with total hospital:

$$\frac{(4,523 \times 100)}{7,201} = 62.81\%$$

Complication rate:

$$\frac{(125 \times 100)}{4,523} = 2.76\%$$

Nosocomial infection rate:

$$\frac{(78 \times 100)}{4,523} = 1.72\%$$

Medicine service gross death rate:

$$\frac{(60 \times 100)}{4{,}523} = 1.33\%$$

Percentage of patients with:

Medicare:

$$\frac{(905 \times 100)}{4{,}523} = 20.01\%$$

Medicaid:

$$\frac{(812 \times 100)}{4{,}523} = 17.95\%$$

Third-party insurance:

$$\frac{(2{,}126 \times 100)}{4{,}523} = 47.00\%$$

Self-pay:

$$\frac{(680 \times 100)}{4{,}523} = 15.03\%$$

Percentage of patients with:

Cancer:

$$\frac{(986 \times 100)}{4{,}523} = 21.80\%$$

Diabetes and its complications:

$$\frac{(625 \times 100)}{4{,}523} = 13.82\%$$

HIV/AIDS:

$$\frac{(123 \times 100)}{4{,}523} = 2.72\%$$

Myocardial infarction:

$$\frac{(450 \times 100)}{4{,}523} = 9.95\%$$

Asthma:

$$\frac{(267 \times 100)}{4{,}523} = 5.90\%$$

Substance abuse:

$$\frac{(98 \times 100)}{4{,}523} = 2.17\%$$

Chapter 9

Exercise 9.1

1. Total annual compensation/Total annual productivity

$$\frac{\$27,040}{312,000} = 0.087 = 0.9 \text{ or 9 cents per line.}$$

2. $\dfrac{\$20,800}{234,000} = 0.089 = 0.9$ or 9 cents per line.

3. a. Transcriptionist who produces 1,000 lines per day:

$$\frac{\$24,960}{260,000} = 0.096 \text{ or 10 cents per line}$$

Transcriptionist who produces 1,200 lines per day:

$$\frac{\$24,960}{312,000} = 0.08 = 8 \text{ cents per line}$$

b. Both make $12.00 per hour, but one produces 1,000 and one produces 1,200 lines per day. As the production increases, the labor unit cost decreases.

c. Transcriptionist who produces 1,000 per day:

$$\frac{\$27,040}{260,000} = 0.10 \text{ or 10 cents per line}$$

Transcriptionist who produces 1,100 per day

$$\frac{\$27,040}{286,000} = 0.09 \text{ or 9 cents per line}$$

d. Total compensation/total productivity

The total annual salaries for the eight transcriptionists = $211,120.

The total medical transcriptionist's annual productivity = 2,184,000 lines per year.

The unit cost = $211,120/2,184,000 = 0.97 or 10 cents per line

Exercise 9.3

1. Postage: $\dfrac{\$465}{542} = \$0.84$ per request

    Service contract: $\dfrac{\$216}{542} = 0.398 = \$0.40$ per request

    Equipment: $\dfrac{\$135}{542} = 0.249 = \$0.25$ per request

    Supplies: $\dfrac{\$110}{542} = \$0.20$ per request

    Wages: $\$11.00 \times 2{,}080 = \$22{,}880$ annual salary

    $\dfrac{\$22{,}880}{12} = \$1{,}906.66$

    $\dfrac{\$1{,}906.66}{542} = 3.5217 = \$3.52$

2. Monthly cost: $\$0.84 + \$0.40 + \$0.25 + \$0.20 + \$3.52 = \$5.21$ per request $\times 542$ requests $= \$2{,}823.82$

3. $\$2{,}823.82 - \$1{,}500.00 = \$1{,}323.82$

Exercise 9.5

Telephone requests: $\$3.75 \times 150 = \$562.50$

Online Appointment Request Form: $\$150.00 \times 150 = \$225.00$

Cost savings: $\$562.50 - \$225.00 = \$337.50$ or $\$2.25$ per appointment

Exercise 9.7

Department	Week #1	Week #2	Week #3	Week #4	Total	Proportion
Lab	27	34	48	54	**163**	**0.27**
Radiology	15	21	26	42	**104**	**0.17**
Pathology	25	26	28	31	**110**	**0.18**
Nursing	17	22	36	41	**116**	**0.19**
Physical therapy	5	4	2	12	**23**	**0.04**
Miscellaneous	20	21	22	26	**89**	**0.15**
Totals	**109**	**128**	**162**	**206**	**605**	**1.0**

Exercise 9.9

1. 5,000 inpatient records $\times$ 30 pages $= 150{,}000$

    2,000 outpatient records $\times$ 4 pages $= 8{,}000$

    1,500 ED records $\times$ 3 $= 4{,}500$

    $\dfrac{(150{,}000 + 8{,}000 + 4{,}000)}{1{,}500} = 108.0$ days

2. 3.6 FTEs needed.

$$\frac{108}{30} = 3.6$$

or

$$\frac{162,000}{30 \text{ days}} = 5,400 \text{ pages needing to be scanned}$$

$$\frac{5,400}{1,500} = 3.6 \text{ FTEs needed}$$

3. a. Coder A: $\dfrac{(425 \times 100)}{1,300} = 32.69\%$

    Coder B: $\dfrac{(502 \times 100)}{1,300} = 38.62\%$

    Coder C: $\dfrac{(373 \times 100)}{1,300} = 28.69\%$

  b. Coder A: $\dfrac{425}{21} = 20.24$

    Coder B: $\dfrac{502}{21} = 23.90$

    Coder C: $\dfrac{373}{21} = 17.76$

  c. Coder A: $\dfrac{20.24}{8} = 2.53$

    Coder B: $\dfrac{23.90}{8} = 2.99$

    Coder C: $\dfrac{17.76}{8} = 2.22$

  d. Coder A: $\dfrac{60}{2.53} = 23.72$

    Coder B: $\dfrac{60}{2.99} = 20.07$

    Coder C: $\dfrac{60}{2.22} = 27.03$

  e. Coder A: $\dfrac{(4 \times 100)}{425} = 0.94\%$

    Coder B: $\dfrac{(3 \times 100)}{502} = 0.60\%$

    Coder C: $\dfrac{(11 \times 100)}{373} = 2.95\%$

Exercise 9.11

1. The gross death rate is calculated by dividing the total number of deaths by the total number of discharges.

$$\frac{((7+2)\times100)}{650}=1.38\%$$

This statistic may be more meaningful to administration or the medical staff than the whole number of 1 percent. Death rates often are calculated to the second decimal place.

2. $\dfrac{(2\times100)}{9}=22.22\%$

3. MS-DRG 844, Other myeloprolific disorder or poorly differentiated neoplasm diagnosis with complication or comorbidity has an ALOS of 23 days.

4. FRP: $\dfrac{(5\times100)}{75}=6.67\%$

   GI: $\dfrac{(5\times100)}{27}=18.52\%$

   MED: $\dfrac{(59\times100)}{511}=11.55\%$

   MON: $\dfrac{(26\times100)}{67}=38.81\%$

   NB: $\dfrac{(1\times100)}{129}=0.78\%$

   NPH: $\dfrac{(42\times100)}{162}=25.93\%$

   ORS: $\dfrac{(2\times100)}{14}=14.29\%$

   PED: $\dfrac{(1\times100)}{55}=1.82\%$

   THS: $\dfrac{(3\times100)}{37}=8.11\%$

   VSS: $\dfrac{(1\times100)}{26}=3.85\%$

   Overall rate: $\dfrac{(188\times100)}{2,046}=9.19\%$

5. Case-mix—All financial classes for Fiscal year:

$$\frac{6831.0912}{3,230} = 2.1149$$

Case-mix—All financial classes for Month End 10/20XX:

$$\frac{3396.8017}{1,626} = 2.0891$$

Case-mix—Medicare only for Month End 10/20XX:

$$\frac{1364.1506}{658} = 2.0732$$

There were 1,367 Medicare discharges year-to-date. This report was calculated for month end October.

Chapter 10

Exercise 10.1

1. True

2. 27, 35, 54, 56, 65, 74, 75, 76, 77, 84, 86, 88, 89, 91, 92, 93, 94, 95, 96, 97, 99, 100

$$\frac{(11 \times 100)}{22} = 50\text{th percentile}$$

Exercise 10.3

1. The range for the data may be expressed as 17 (the difference) or as 1 to 18 (quoting the smallest and largest values); however, keep in mind that in mathematics, the range is usually expressed as one value.

2. a. 3 to 15 or 12

   b. –4 to 15 or 19

   c. 42 to 127 or 85

3. 3 + 22 = 25

4. 107 – 54 = 53

5. 227 – 127 = 100

Chapter 11

Exercise 11.1

1. This is an example of the nominal data or scale. In the nominal scale of measurement, you are only allowed to examine whether the data are equal to some particular value or to count the number of occurrences of each value. For example, gender is a nominal scale variable. You can examine whether the gender of a person is female or to count the number of males in a sample.

2. This is an example of ordinal scale. Ordinal data are types of data where the values are in ordered categories. On the ordinal scale, the order of the numbers is meaningful, not the number itself. This is because the intervals or distance between categories are not necessarily equal.

3. No, because temperature is an interval scale of measurement and the zero on the scale does not represent the absence of the thing being measured. Interval measurement ratios do not make sense: 80 degrees is not twice as hot as 40 degrees (although the attribute value is twice as large).

4. Yes, because this is an example of ratio scale of measurement. There is a zero point; that is you can have zero patients.

5. This is an example of an ordinal scale of measurement. Measurements with ordinal scales are ordered in the sense that higher numbers represent higher values. However, the intervals between the numbers are not necessarily equal. For example, on the five-point rating scale measuring correct information given by the clerk, the difference between a rating of 2 and a rating of 3 may not represent the same difference as the difference between a rating of 4 and a rating of 5.

6. The scales of these variables would be: b. nominal, ratio, ordinal, ordinal. The first question, whether the mothers drank, is answered yes or no. In the nominal scale, observations are organized into categories. The birth weight of the baby is a ratio scale, which has a defined unit of measure, a real zero point, and equal intervals between successive values. The Apgar scores at one minute and at five minutes are examples of ordinal data.

Exercise 11.3

Community Hospital
Ages of Patients with Colon Cancer
Annual Statistics 20XX

Ages	No. of Patients	Proportion
≤ 30	3	**0.01**
31–40	12	**0.06**
41–50	18	**0.09**
51–60	60	**0.29**
61–70	65	**0.32**
70+	48	**0.23**

Exercise 11.5

1.

2.

3.

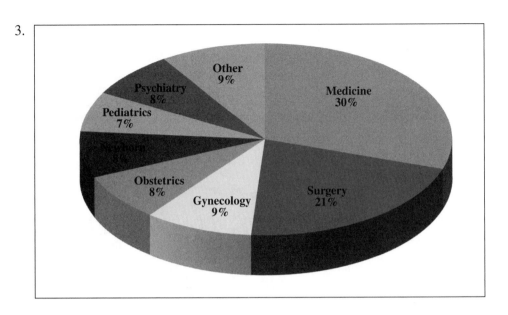

4.

LENGTH OF STAY DISTRIBUTION

	PATIENTS	% CASES
SAME DAY	114	1.7
1 DAY	755	11.3
2–4 DAYS	1,343	20.2
5–7 DAYS	1,555	23.3
8–14 DAYS	1,469	22.0
15–42 DAYS	1,217	18.3
43+ DAYS	210	3.2
Total	6,663	100.0

Exercise 11.7

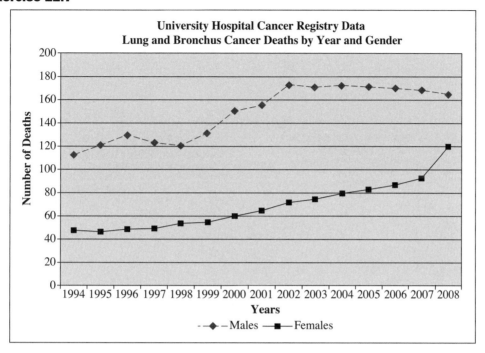

Chapter 12

Exercise 12.1

Fail to reject the null hypothesis, or not statistically significant at the .05 level. This is because there is a greater than 5% chance that the null hypothesis is correct.

Index